"Richard Tedeschi and Bret Moore's *The Posttraumatic Growth Workbook* is a gift to people suffering from loss, grief, and trauma. These useful exercises and helpful—and *hopeful*—readings will not only assist you as you cope with loss, but, more importantly, will help you to continue to grow, despite loss and grief."

— **Rev. Kenneth J. Doka, PhD**, professor at the College of New Rochelle
Graduate School, senior consultant for the Hospice Foundation of America,
and author of *Grief is a Journey*

"If there were no trauma, there would be no posttraumatic growth. When trauma happens, a new path begins. This path may be full of sorrow and despair, but we are not alone. In spite of trauma, we can grow as people. This book offers the key to unlocking our true potential."

— **Kanako Taku**, certified clinical psychologist in Japan, and associate professor
in the psychology department at Oakland University

"We see the suffering and results of over fifteen years of war in Iraq and Afghanistan on a daily basis at Boulder Crest Retreat for Military and Veteran Wellness. We also see the amount of strength that exists in military families. If there is one community in our nation that can achieve posttraumatic growth, it is the combat veteran who was forged on the anvil of adversity, and the military family that endured the long and stressful deployments. This workbook is a must for our brothers and sisters who have witnessed the worst that humanity has to offer—war."

— **Ken Falke**, retired US Navy Bomb Disposal specialist, philanthropist, and
founder of the EOD Warrior Foundation and Boulder Crest Retreat for Military
and Veteran Wellness

T0304931

The
Posttraumatic
Growth
Workbook

Coming Through Trauma
Wiser, Stronger,
and More Resilient

Richard G. Tedeschi, PhD
Bret A. Moore, PsyD, ABPP

New Harbinger Publications, Inc.

Publisher's Note

This publication is designed to provide accurate and authoritative information in regard to the subject matter covered. It is sold with the understanding that the publisher is not engaged in rendering psychological, financial, legal, or other professional services. If expert assistance or counseling is needed, the services of a competent professional should be sought.

NEW HARBINGER PUBLICATIONS is a registered trademark of New Harbinger Publications, Inc.

New Harbinger Publications is an employee-owned company

Copyright © 2016 by Richard G. Tedeschi and Bret A. Moore
New Harbinger Publications, Inc.
5720 Shattuck Avenue
Oakland, CA 94609
www.newharbinger.com

Cover design by Amy Shoup

Acquired by Melissa Kirk

Edited by Brady Kahn

All Rights Reserved

Library of Congress Cataloging-in-Publication Data on file

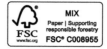

Printed in the United States of America

26   25   24

10   9   8   7   6

To Joan, Michael, and Anna Caroline, for all your enthusiasm for life.

—RGT

To Lori and Kaitlyn, for your patience, understanding, and unconditional love.

—BAM

We would like to dedicate this book to the thousands of men, women, and children whom we have had the pleasure to serve over our collective fifty years of practice. Their experiences, stories, and lives have done much to shape who we are and how we see the world today.

—RGT and BAM

Contents

Acknowledgments

Without the support of many people in our lives, this book would not be possible. We would like to thank our families for their encouragement and patience. The trauma survivors to whom we have been companions over the years have been the greatest source of knowledge and inspiration for us. We wish to especially recognize the work on developing the concept of posttraumatic growth, contributed over many years, by Lawrence Calhoun, and the many other colleagues and students who have also played important roles in developing this field. We are indebted to Dr. Matthew Whalley of Psychology Tools for reminding us of the power found within simple techniques. We are grateful for the professionalism and dedication of the publishing staff of New Harbinger, specifically Brady Kahn, who has been masterful in editing this book. And last, we would like to thank Ken Falke, Josh Goldberg, and all the staff of Boulder Crest Retreat. Their mission and dedication inspire and cause us to constantly refine our thinking and apply our ideas in new ways.

Introduction

At the time of our writing this book, the American military has taken virtually all of its troops out of Afghanistan and Iraq, which would appear to close a chapter on a traumatic period in American life that began on September 11, 2001. But 9/11 and the ensuing combat were not the only traumas with which the American public became intimately familiar. Also in the news were natural disasters such as Hurricane Katrina and Hurricane Sandy. More difficult to understand is the horror committed by humans. In San Bernardino, California, a radicalized couple killed fourteen innocent people enjoying a holiday party and wounded twenty-one others. And none of us will ever forget the tragic slaughter of twenty first-graders and six adults at Sandy Hook Elementary School in Newtown, Connecticut. However, it doesn't stop there. There are the stories of clergy sexually abusing children. The country endured a major economic recession that dashed the plans of many and put thousands of Americans out of their homes. There is the Ebola epidemic in West Africa. And many individuals have personal traumas that never make the news but are just as emotionally wrenching—battles with terrible illnesses, unemployment, family disruption, loss, and grief.

Because of the attention paid to trauma in the media, Americans have become increasingly familiar with the problem of post-traumatic stress disorder (PTSD), an often chronic and disabling psychological condition that wreaks havoc on those who suffer from it as well as on their loved ones. Even though PTSD is a response that can be linked to a variety of traumatic experiences, such as rape, car accidents, and natural disasters, most people relate this syndrome to the experience of combat veterans. But anyone who is confronted with an experience that is physically or emotionally threatening can develop PTSD or some symptoms of it.

There are a number of good books already available to help people cope with the symptoms and experience of trauma, recover from trauma, and become stronger. Like other books on trauma recovery, this book is for people who have faced or are continuing to face adversity in their lives and are looking for ways to navigate it successfully. But this book takes trauma survivors beyond simply learning how to cope better. This book is designed for those who wish to go beyond being resilient, to experience meaningful personal growth and perhaps radical transformation in the aftermath of a trauma. We will give you the tools to thrive, grow, and transform yourself. As one trauma survivor told us, "Why waste this traumatic experience on just getting back to who I was?" Consider the following story.

Joe had wanted to join the Army as far back as he could remember. He got the chance when he turned eighteen, only two weeks after finishing high school. Joe was from a small town in Mississippi and grew up in a lower-middle class family. He was the oldest of four boys, all of whom had visions of escaping their small town existence with the help of the military. Joe's mother was a kind and caring woman. A devout Christian, she was heavily involved in the church, which meant Joe and his brothers were as well. His father was a different story. Although not a physically abusive man, Joe's dad was prone to angry outbursts that could easily be classified as emotional abuse. These outbursts were most prominent when he was drinking, which happened frequently. His father's drinking and anger drove a wedge between his father and him at an early age. They fought constantly. Being the oldest, Joe found himself acting as a buffer between his dad and the rest of the family. He despised his dad for putting him in this position. Things came to a head the night before Joe was scheduled to leave for basic training. During a drunken episode, Joe's father told him that he was a deserter and a coward for leaving the family. Joe's last words to his father were "I hate you and hope you die."

The week before Joe was set to deploy to Iraq, he received a call from his father. The last time he had heard from him was two years earlier, the night before he had left for the Army. When Joe's father disclosed that he had been diagnosed with cancer, Joe was surprised by his own reaction. Although he felt sad, his anger toward his dad seemed to somehow blunt his reaction to the news. It's not that he didn't care; he just wasn't devastated like he thought he should be. The phone call ended with a promise by Joe to stay in touch throughout his deployment.

Joe thrived in the combat zone. He was part of a close-knit team and enjoyed his work. Most days he spent walking through neighborhoods searching for suspected terrorists. Then one day, about five months into his deployment, things changed for him. On a routine patrol in a "friendly" neighborhood, Joe's unit came under attack, and over one-third of his unit was injured, including Joe and a buddy. Joe received relatively minor shrapnel injuries to both of his legs and suffered a dislocated shoulder. His buddy wasn't so lucky. The roadside bomb that caused Joe's injuries severed both of his friend's legs, and he later died.

Joe struggled after his friend's death. He had problems with sleep, suffering from constant nightmares. He couldn't stop thinking about what had happened to his friend and how he wished he could somehow have saved him. He became depressed and withdrawn. After a while, he came to this realization: "I'd been so concerned about how I might have saved Randy that I ignored something else. I just miss the guy. I've had lots of friends but no one like him. Maybe it's because of all we went through together, but it was more than that. We just knew what the other was thinking. He was more a brother to me than my real brothers have ever been. I guess I should be grieving, and I have just been kicking myself around, feeling guilty. Now, I think it's selfish. I think I have been thinking more about myself than honoring him—what a great guy he was, how he always backed me up. I don't know if he knew that's what I thought of him. I guess you always think you have plenty of time."

Thinking this way led Joe to see the importance of relationships and how hard it is to predict how long people will be in your life: "I'm wondering now how I'll feel when my father is gone. We've had a crappy relationship for years. I guess I've just chalked it up as a waste. I started to think about how I'll feel about all this in years to come. I already knew there was something not right about my reaction to my dad's cancer. I knew it was a weird reaction. I was numb to it. I knew I would like to feel differently, but I didn't know how to get there, and part of me was so angry and hurt by him, I didn't want to. It was easy to feel the loss of Randy because we were all good with each other, but I couldn't feel what it would be like to lose my dad. This whole thing with the war and loss and all, it forced me to deal with stuff that maybe I would never have gotten to. I don't know. It all forced my hand?"

Joe describes how trauma can be a window into a new perspective on how you are living your life. For Joe, there was more to it than he'd imagined.

Ultimately, Joe's anger toward his father seemed to give way to compassion. In one week, Joe called his father on two separate occasions. Their conversations focused on how his father was doing and on how Joe would like to mend their relationship. He apologized for telling his father that he hated him and expressed how ashamed he was for telling him that he wished he would die. After all these years, a caring, open, and respectful relationship between Joe and his father began to form.

This book is about the kind of growth that can happen in the aftermath of trauma, as Joe discovered. We refer to this process as *posttraumatic growth*, or PTG. One of us, Rich, coined this term in the early 1990s, and together with his colleague Lawrence Calhoun, Rich has been at the forefront of gaining an understanding of this process and gathering research on how and why it occurs. The basic concept is that positive personal transformation can occur in the aftermath of trauma. The stories of survivors of combat, rape, cancer, natural disaster, and other traumas are often not only about psychological suffering but also about some remarkably positive changes that these survivors have experienced following trauma. Their stories are often stories of discovery and a sense of newfound meaning and purpose.

In this book, you will find ways in which you can enhance your chances of strengthening yourself through the great pain of loss or trauma. This book will show you how to use your struggles with life's losses and tragedies to develop in ways that might not have been possible without them.

The concept of posttraumatic growth has been recognized for centuries. From the ancient Greeks to today, tragedy has been a common theme in many great works of literature. It is also an essential ingredient in soap operas, movies, novels, and the stories people love. Perhaps the enduring appeal of these stories for most of us is that they teach the lessons of suffering without our having to experience the pain directly. The great religions of the world also teach that suffering can lead to wisdom. In the Judeo-Christian tradition, stories of suffering are viewed as lessons. The story of Job is one of the most famous examples of human suffering. The central teaching of the New Testament is that without the tragedy of the cross, humans would forever remain unconnected to God. Reinhold Niebuhr, the author of the Serenity Prayer, has pointed out that Christianity changes tragedy into something that is not tragedy, and this is clearly the message of the resurrection of Christ. Other religions also view suffering as a path toward goodness. Certain tenets of Islam suggest that suffering is something to be welcomed, because it is seen as instrumental in the purposes of God. As a Muslim colleague once said, "If you suffer, it means that you have been especially chosen by

God." Buddhism directs people to approach suffering and learn from it rather than avoid pain, and the Four Noble Truths are a guide to this process.

For most people, the lessons of religion or the stories of transformation found in literature exist in the background, and life just sort of rattles on. But a major loss or, if you are lucky, the mere threat of a major loss, can shake you out of your complacent routine. As the shock of the trauma wears off, you can experience important positive changes. We have found that these changes vary from person to person, but there are some common themes. For example, you may greet each new day with greater appreciation. You may become more aware of the strength in yourself that has enabled you to manage a difficult life situation. As a survivor of trauma, you may have a greater appreciation for how much your loved ones and others care about you. You may have begun to explore new opportunities or life paths. Perhaps your understanding of spiritual matters has changed. This book will explore these kinds of changes. We will provide you with some practical ways to live in the aftermath of trauma so that you may gain the most from your experience.

It is possible. The numbers vary widely, but on average research studies show that 60 percent of people who experience trauma also report posttraumatic growth (Calhoun and Tedeschi 2006). In the aftermath of a wide range of traumatic events, many people are able to find some benefit. These events include the onset of physical disability, terminal illness, divorce, bereavement, natural and man-made disasters, rape, sexual abuse, accidents, combat, or the onset of a child's serious illness or disability. If you have experienced such an event and wish to respond in a way that makes this a positive turning point in your life, be assured that this experience is possible for you. This book will help you find a new direction.

You may wonder, what if I have PTSD? How can I move toward posttraumatic growth if I am struggling with PTSD? The truth is that the same challenges that create PTSD also set the stage for a psychological rebirth. In the aftermath of trauma, what was once an understandable reality has now become something that is mystifying. You have difficulty navigating the strange new life you find yourself living. This difficulty produces the classic symptoms of PTSD: a self-protective posture toward life that is essentially automatic, treating the world as an unsafe place. Being easily startled, having nightmares, feeling emotionally numb, having flashbacks to traumatic events, and feeling mistrustful are all part of this self-protective reaction. But these shocking challenges to the usual way of living can also set in motion an exploration of new ways of living that becomes posttraumatic growth. In fact, some people may experience symptoms of PTSD and posttraumatic growth at the same time. This is one of the paradoxes of posttraumatic growth.

We also want to emphasize that posttraumatic growth is usually experienced without the help of psychologists or other mental health professionals. Just as the symptoms of PTSD are naturally occurring reactions to the dire threats of trauma and often remit without the help of psychiatric professionals, posttraumatic growth is a naturally occurring process of healing and growth that can happen in the weeks, months, and years following trauma. Both PTSD and PTG are natural responses of the mind to the injury of trauma. We therefore speak of *post-traumatic stress injuries* (PTSI) that produce symptoms and also set in motion natural growth processes. We like to use the word "injuries" to emphasize that the reactions that have been called PTSD have a basis in a natural response to extraordinary circumstances. This idea is also part of the new thinking about trauma response and posttraumatic growth.

Just as injuries heal naturally and growth occurs naturally, there are circumstances that hinder healing and growth and circumstances that facilitate it. In this book, we describe what can be done to facilitate healing from PTSI. We describe what trauma survivors can do to help themselves and what people who care for them can do to facilitate the best outcomes in the aftermath of trauma.

This workbook can help you move toward personal change and development. Unfortunately, this process is not something that can be reduced to an easy formula, and we do not want you to be discouraged by the difficulty of the process. Stick with the workbook. Be assured that if you want to take your stressful or traumatic situation and use it as a turning point for personal growth, we can provide you with a way forward. Most people who face stressful or traumatic events are first concerned with wanting to feel better. They are focused on literally surviving after what has happened to them. Some people think that life is not worth living and may even consider suicide. Given this emotional turmoil, the period just after a trauma is usually not a good time to be thinking about growth. You will probably need some time before growth becomes a possibility. At first you need to focus on your basic needs. A homeless person who does not have food or water, adequate clothing, or shelter is not quite ready to begin college, start a career, or foster a budding intimate relationship. Similarly, the basic needs of the trauma survivor, managing intense emotions and life disruption, must be addressed first.

There are a small number of people who do think of growth very early on. Rich recalls a husband and wife, who upon learning that their teenage son was killed in an auto accident, said to each other within a few hours of the event, "This is too horrible a thing to let it be for nothing. We have to make something worthwhile come from this. Otherwise, our son will have died for nothing." When you are ready for growth will depend on how you respond to trauma. As you are reading this book, it may have been years since you experienced a trauma, or conversely, you may still be suffering and perhaps have severe health problems or injuries. Coauthor Bret has worked with many military service members whose injuries represented a daily challenge but for whom growth was still possible.

We want to add that even though posttraumatic growth provides relief from stressful and traumatic events, growth does not make everything better. Many years ago, in her book entitled *Necessary Losses*, Judith Viorst described the perspective that Rabbi Harold Kushner took on the death of his teenage son. Kushner realized that he had changed in many important ways after his son's death: he had become a more empathic and effective rabbi; he had experienced a deepening of his spiritual side. But he also said that he would trade all of that in if he could just have his son back. No amount of growth can completely undo the pain of such a personal loss.

You may still suffer from what has happened to you. Growth will not put an end to all your suffering. However, it may make it easier to bear, because it will become clear that your suffering has not been entirely in vain. There is more to the trauma than the loss or the misery. None of us should be naive about these situations, however. Traumas themselves are never good things, and we do not recommend trauma as a pathway to growth. A misunderstanding about our intentions has led to some angry and misguided responses to us. Rich has received letters from people who have said, "I can't believe you are saying that sending our sons and daughters off to war to get blown up is a good thing for them!" Of course, we are saying no such thing. But given the fact that trauma is a harsh reality of life for so many, how can we encourage the best possible ways to deal with trauma and move forward in life? Ignoring trauma's existence is certainly unhelpful.

Another point to make is that not everyone experiences growth. We do not claim that everyone can. Although growth is commonplace, it is not universal. In some cases, people who experience no posttraumatic growth likewise have experienced little distress following a trauma. Their system of core beliefs allows them to understand what is happening, and they do not have to reconsider what they already know. They are able to get back to their previous way of living without much difficulty. These are the most resilient people. They have a remarkable ability to bounce back. Sometimes these people may have experienced very difficult lives growing up. As a result, they feel that the most recent stressful life experience is more of the same. They may have already learned the lessons of suffering. They have learned that life is hard and full of tragedy. But if trauma has rocked you, and you have not felt resilient, this book will help you change so you feel more resilient in the future. Posttraumatic growth is a pathway to resilience.

As you progress through this workbook, you will meet others who are already on this journey. Their stories are not about despair and hopelessness but about lives made richer and deeper in meaning through posttraumatic growth. We highlight the important tools and methods these trauma survivors used. We draw on our experience as clinical psychologists, educators, and researchers in the areas of trauma, coping, and growth to help you understand the process of posttraumatic growth and how to generate this process in your own life and perhaps in the lives of others. We hope that you will find the stories in this book both comforting and transformative.

One more concept we introduce is *expert companionship*, an idea developed by Rich to help trauma survivors find the support from others that they need to grow. We discuss how you can identify expert companions for yourself and how you can become an expert companion for others. Expert companions are not necessarily professionals and, in fact, are more likely to be friends and family members. You may find it difficult to locate an expert companion, and we encourage you to look in some unlikely places. We are also aware that many of our readers may be friends and family members of trauma survivors, so we will spend some time talking about how to be an expert companion. We describe such characteristics as patience and an ability to join in the perspective of the trauma survivor while noticing and expressing other possibilities for growth.

We have written this book to be accessible and inspirational not only to those who are struggling with trauma and those who are trying to support a loved one who is struggling but also to anyone who is interested in finding greater meaning and purpose. To get the most out of this book, you will need to do more than just read it. This workbook is organized around a series of psychological tasks or exercises that are designed to reveal the seeds of posttraumatic growth in your experience and to nurture them. Again, some of these exercises might be emotionally difficult to do, especially if your trauma is quite recent. You may find that this is a book to start now and return to later. After more time has passed, you may be better able to respond to some of the challenges we present. You may want to keep a blank journal close to hand as you go through this workbook, both to give yourself additional space to complete the exercises or try them again and to record your thoughts about your journey.

We have spent our entire professional lives—over fifty years between the two of us—working with trauma survivors: Bret with active duty soldiers, including nearly two and a half years in Iraq, and Rich with bereaved parents and a variety of other trauma survivors in Charlotte, North Carolina. We have both written many books for our professional colleagues about this work, and Bret has written books for veterans on postcombat adjustment. This is our first book written especially for trauma survivors, and we are pleased to speak directly to you. One thing that we have kept in mind while writing is that most of our information comes from the people we have tried to help. Who has informed us the most? For Rich, it is the bereaved parents that he worked with for twenty-five years in a nonprofit bereavement agency. For Bret, as an Army psychologist, it is the active duty soldiers and veterans who have endured terrible combat experiences.

But both of us also have worked with many survivors of other kinds of traumatic events, including cancer, sexual abuse, airplane crashes, divorce, hurricanes, and many other personal trials. These survivors have taught us what it has been like to go through their traumas and what kind of help they needed. We have tried to use what we have learned from them to help you. We hope that you can see the good sense of these brave people in the pages of this book. You will find many places where we quote them. Hearing about their experiences may help you see that you are not alone in your struggles and that others have successfully traveled a similar path.

We hope that by listening to trauma survivors and helping them navigate the aftermath of their own traumas, we have learned how to be good expert companions. We want to share what we have learned with you—the trauma survivor or the person wanting to help. We want to share with you how to discover, and often create, a new way of living that makes the struggle following trauma meaningful and valuable, when the trauma itself may have been simply horrific.

You have likely picked up this book because this idea attracted you. If you are going to have to go through the tragedy and loss of trauma, why not make sure there is also something worthwhile in the end? Back as far as the 1980s, Rich, along with his colleague Lawrence Calhoun at the University of North Carolina at Charlotte, began to listen to the stories of trauma survivors who found themselves on paths of personal growth and transformation. In this workbook, we hope that you will find a pathway to personal transformation as well. We are eager to share with you the wisdom of other trauma survivors, their accomplishments, and the ways we have devised to encourage the process of posttraumatic growth.

Because of the focus on posttraumatic growth, this workbook is different from others that you will find on trauma recovery, post-traumatic stress disorder, and the like. We are not naive about the difficulties of trauma survivors, but we see clearly their possible futures. We hope that as you read, and as you work through the exercises in this workbook and apply them to your life, you will also see a bright future for yourself.

Note: If you're a clinician hoping to use this book with those you treat, you will find a bonus chapter addressing this at http://www.newharbinger.com/34688.

CHAPTER 1

Trauma and Growth

Benjamin Franklin is credited with saying "In this world nothing can be said to be certain, except death and taxes." We would argue another certainty is that at some point, virtually everyone experiences a life event that is traumatic. Such events usually come as surprises, as if we were all immune to what other people experience. Granted, you can structure your daily routine and environment to provide you with some degree of predictability. Each day, you can go to bed and wake at the same time, check e-mails when you first get to work or eat dinner while watching your favorite television show. But in reality, we are all susceptible and vulnerable to the countless unknowns lurking in the different nooks and crannies of life. This is no better exemplified than by how trauma can emerge from these blind spots of life and hit us without warning.

Another certainty is that people respond to trauma differently. The psychological impact on an unsuspecting eighteen-year-old college student who is sexually assaulted while walking to her car in a dark parking garage will be different from the experience of the soldier who nearly dies after his vehicle is hit with a roadside bomb. The college student's sense of safety and security within the world will likely be shattered. She may begin to have difficulty trusting other people or become overwhelmed with anxiety when she goes out in public. The soldier, a professional who has trained for years to deal with adversity, may be "fine" initially but go on to develop terrible nightmares and depression months or even years later. Both have faced terrible psychological and physical assaults. But the symptoms they experience, the personal narrative they tell themselves about what happened, and the trajectory of their recovery will differ. This book will explore why this is true, but for now, the key point to remember is that when faced with traumatic events, including events that may share many similarities, everyone's experience and outcome will be different.

In spite of these differences, however, we all possess the same basic machinery that switches on in response to trauma. The primary goal of this chapter is to provide you with an understanding of this basic human response. Although it may seem illogical, you will learn how your responses to trauma can be both adaptive and protective.

Trauma and Its Effects

It's been estimated that about three-fourths of adults over age sixty-five have been exposed to at least one traumatic event during their lifetime, and depending on the definition of traumatic event, the figure may be even higher (Mills et al. 2011). Traumas include sexual and physical assaults, motor vehicle accidents, serious illnesses, combat, and a host of manmade and natural disasters. Furthermore, we have learned that for many people, other events may be traumatic as well, and it is hard to determine what events will be particularly difficult for an individual. Men experience trauma at a greater rate than women. This may be a result of the disproportionate number of men serving in combat or their tendency to engage in riskier behaviors. Women, however, tend to be more susceptible to developing psychological complications following trauma. This is due to the fact that the traumatic events suffered by women tend to be more severe, chronic, and of a personal nature. For example, sexual assault, especially during childhood, is often a repeated violation and wreaks tremendous emotional damage. Although men certainly experience sexual abuse as children, the reality is that most victims are women. And not uncommonly, men and women may experience multiple traumatic events in their lives, which leads to even greater psychological distress—just as a windshield will maintain its integrity after a single crack from a rock but break down over time with repeated hits (Norris 1992).

Early in his career, Bret learned an important concept as he provided care to soldiers in Iraq: psychological distress following trauma is not an abnormal reaction but rather a normal reaction to an abnormal event. Most anyone who is exposed to an unthinkable psychological or physical injury will struggle to some degree. This is to be expected and should not be thought of as a sickness or illness. This is why it may be useful to think of the difficulties experienced following trauma as a post-traumatic stress injury, as we mentioned in the introduction. PTSI is an obvious and expected reaction to an abnormal event. Most everyone will experience worry, fear, sadness, nightmares, and insomnia after witnessing a tragic car accident, surviving a natural disaster like a tornado, or losing a loved one unexpectedly. Our bodies and minds are knocked out of balance…for a while. Most of us return to normal with time, help from others, and reliance on our own internal strength. It's only when the struggle becomes too great for too long that it becomes something more like post-traumatic stress disorder. But even those who meet the diagnostic criteria for PTSD have suffered an injury to their way of understanding their world, which results in the symptoms that have been called PTSD.

The immediate aftereffects of trauma vary. However, a number of emotional, mental, behavioral, and physical symptoms commonly appear within the initial hours and days following a traumatic event. These are listed in the following chart.

Emotional	Mental	Behavioral	Physical
Feeling alone	Loss of concentration	Withdrawal from others	Aches and pains
Feeling afraid	Disorientation and confusion	Impulsive behavior	Fatigue and tiredness
Anger and frustration	Memory loss	Aggression	Racing heart
Mood swings	Obsessive thoughts	Crying	Nausea and vomiting
Difficulty sleeping	Distractibility	Arguing with loved ones	Shakiness and trembling
Feeling sad	Indecisiveness	Increased sleeping	Headaches
Feeling hopeless	Thoughts about death and dying	Changes in appetite	Numbness and tingling
Helplessness	Racing thoughts	Being easily startled	Diarrhea
Feeling numb		Increased drug or alcohol use	Hot flushes
Anxiety and panic			
Nightmares			
Lack of confidence			

These symptoms are normal immediately following trauma, and in most cases, they will go away after time. This is not to minimize the many and varied effects of trauma but rather to reassure anyone reading this book who has recently experienced a traumatic event—or knows someone who has—that these reactions are to be expected. Information and awareness can be very powerful and therapeutic. In the following exercise, you will identify the symptoms that you experienced after a traumatic event. This exercise will help you normalize the event and its effects as well as identify any symptoms you may be experiencing. Our hope is that many of the symptoms you identify have either gone away or lessened over time. Please pay particular attention to those symptoms you have battled and overcome. It speaks to the strength and resilience you have within you. If some symptoms remain, acknowledge the impact they have on you, but also identify how you manage them on a daily basis. Even though you may feel that you can't manage some of the more difficult ones, the reality is that you have likely developed various coping strategies over time that keep you in the fight to survive and live a satisfying life after trauma.

Being Reluctant or Being Surprised by Your Emotions

Looking at your own reaction to a traumatic event can be difficult. You may find that you become emotional as you recall a traumatic event and write out the details of it. You might feel at some point that your vivid memories of an event make you feel as if you were reliving it. We understand that you may wonder if this is a good idea, as you may feel worse when completing this exercise. If this exercise causes you a great deal of distress, you can certainly stop and reconsider if you are ready to continue. However, one of the things that is most helpful to people who have experienced trauma is to confront it directly. The accompanying distress is not an indication that this is a destructive process. In fact, your distress probably indicates that your rethinking the event will lead to posttraumatic growth.

EXERCISE: Your Reaction to the Traumatic Event

First write out a brief narrative about a past traumatic event. Which event you choose is up to you. Even if you have experienced repeated trauma, there will be one or two events that stand out more than others. In our clinical work, we have found, especially in those who have suffered many repeated traumas, that it's best to start with the trauma that has had the biggest effect on you. If you aren't sure which one that is, it may be helpful to ask yourself, *Which event do I spend the most time thinking about?* Or if you tell yourself, *If event X had not happened, my life would be different*, then event X would be a good place to start. If you are still not sure which past traumatic event to choose, just choose the most recent one or the one that is most vivid. There really is no right or wrong choice. Plus, if you find this exercise helpful, you can use it to explore other past traumatic events.

Describe the traumatic event in as much detail as possible, and use extra space by writing in your journal, if necessary.

_____

_____

_____

_____

After you have described the trauma, identify any emotional, mental, behavioral, or physical symptoms you experienced in the immediate aftermath or over a long time afterward. You can refer to the chart that appeared earlier in this chapter for a list of possibilities. Note whether or not the symptoms persist. If the symptoms have gone away, estimate how long it took for them to disappear. And finally, if symptoms have gone away or even lessened in severity, identify what you did to overcome them. If a symptom is still present, you may also write about how you continue to cope with it. Write in the space provided or in your journal if you need more room.

Emotional symptoms:

1. _____

Is the symptom still present? If no, how long did it take to go away? How did you cope and overcome it? If still present, how do you cope with the symptom now?

_____

_____

2. _____

Is the symptom still present? If no, how long did it take to go away? How did you cope and overcome it? If still present, how do you cope with the symptom now?

_____

_____

3. _____

Is the symptom still present? If no, how long did it take to go away? How did you cope and overcome it? If still present, how do you cope with the symptom now?

_____

_____

Mental symptoms:

1. _____

Is the symptom still present? If no, how long did it take to go away? How did you cope and overcome it? If still present, how do you cope with the symptom now?

_____

_____

2. _____

Is the symptom still present? If no, how long did it take to go away? How did you cope and overcome it? If still present, how do you cope with the symptom now?

_____

_____

3. _____

Is the symptom still present? If no, how long did it take to go away? How did you cope and overcome it? If still present, how do you cope with the symptom now?

_____

_____

Behavioral symptoms:

1. _____

Is the symptom still present? If no, how long did it take to go away? How did you cope and overcome it? If still present, how do you cope with the symptom now?

_____

_____

2. _____

Is the symptom still present? If no, how long did it take to go away? How did you cope and overcome it? If still present, how do you cope with the symptom now?

_____

_____

3. _____

Is the symptom still present? If no, how long did it take to go away? How did you cope and overcome it? If still present, how do you cope with the symptom now?

_____

_____

Physical symptoms:

1. _____

Is the symptom still present? If no, how long did it take to go away? How did you cope and overcome it? If still present, how do you cope with the symptom now?

_____

_____

2. _____

Is the symptom still present? If no, how long did it take to go away? How did you cope and overcome it? If still present, how do you cope with the symptom now?

_____

_____

3. _____

Is the symptom still present? If no, how long did it take to go away? How did you cope and overcome it? If still present, how do you cope with the symptom now?

_____

_____

After completing this exercise, take a few minutes to reflect on what it was like for you and how you feel. An exercise like this is easy for some people while emotionally draining for others. If you have a tendency to distance yourself from your emotions (which many trauma survivors do), you may have whipped through it as if checking off items on a grocery list. If this is the case, consider returning to the exercise and focusing on your feelings that are tied to the event. If you are someone who tends to get deeply emotionally invested and feel overwhelmed, now would be a good time to take a break from the book and talk with someone you trust, take a walk, or sit quietly. If you are alone, acknowledge your emotions and let them pass through your mind without any judgment or labels.

_____

The Useful Side of Trauma

One last point we'd like to make about trauma is that it can be useful to a degree. Yes, believe it or not, trauma can serve an adaptive and protective purpose. Take Alison, for example. As a newly licensed teenage driver, she had a habit of driving too fast and sometimes outright recklessly. One evening while driving home from a friend's house, she entered a curve too fast and crashed into a guardrail. The force of the impact flipped her car over the rail, and she landed twenty feet below in a creek bed. Although Alison suffered physical injuries that were not life threatening, the wreck had a tremendous psychological impact on her for many months. Specifically, she became anxious approaching curves and bridges whenever she drove anywhere. Although the anxiety was not severe enough to stop her from driving, it did prompt her to slow down when she drove, and she became a more conscientious and safer driver. In fact, during her senior year of high school, she travelled around to local schools to talk with other students about the importance of driving safely.

Alison's story highlights the complexity of the psychological impact of trauma. Even within the darkness and despair that can follow trauma, if you look hard enough, it's possible to see some positive aspect to it. However, we are far from trying to sell you on a "when life gives you lemons, make lemonade" or "turn that frown upside down" type of psychology. The human psyche is more complex than that. We are, instead, trying to make you aware that you don't have to take a fatalistic view of trauma. There can be more than a glimmer of light in the darkness. And as you will learn in this book, something much more positive can come from the aftermath of trauma if you approach this time with care and deliberate action.

What Is Post-Traumatic Stress Disorder?

When the psychological and physiological effects of trauma continue for months after the event and cause significant disruption in your work, family, social, and/or spiritual life, a diagnosis of post-traumatic stress disorder may be diagnosed by a mental health professional. PTSD develops after exposure to a traumatic event and includes psychological and behavioral symptoms such as reexperiencing the trauma through flashbacks or nightmares, avoidance of reminders of the trauma, and being easily startled. The following chart lists the clinical symptoms of PTSD (American Psychiatric Association 2013).

Intrusive Sympoms	Avoidance Symptoms	Negative Thoughts and Mood	Arousal and Activity
Pervasive and intrusive memories	Avoidance of trauma-related thoughts, memories, or feelings	Trauma-related memory problems	Irritable, angry, or aggressive behavior
Nightmares	Avoidance of reminders of the event (people, places, things)	Negative beliefs and expectations about self, others, and the world	Reckless behavior
Flashbacks/ dissociation		Persistent blaming of self or other people	Always on guard
Extreme distress associated with reminders of the event		Negative and distressing emotions	Easily startled
Increased physiological reaction to reminders of the event		Loss of interest and pleasure in things	Difficulty concentrating
		Feeling disconnected from others	Difficulty falling and staying asleep
		Lack of positive emotions	

Roughly one in twelve (or 8 percent) of Americans will develop PTSD at some point in their lives, with some groups experiencing higher rates (Kilpatrick et al. 2013). Estimates of PTSD in veterans are as high as 30 percent. And because of a variety of factors, such as the often chronic and personal nature of traumatic events, women are approximately twice as likely as men to develop the disorder (Nebraska Department of Veterans' Affairs 2007).

There are a number of factors that influence whether or not someone develops PTSD. These factors are usually referred to as *risk*, *protective*, and *maintenance* factors. The following list of examples was largely adapted from Johnson and Thompson (2008) and Freeman and Freeman (2009).

Risk factors for PTSD include those things that make you more likely to develop the disorder:

- Lower financial and educational status

- Experiencing a mental illness in the past

- Suffering a physical injury

- Seeing people hurt, killed, or maimed

- Feeling a sense of helplessness, horror, or fear after the trauma

- Having little or no support from family, friends, or the community

- Managing additional stress, such as the death of a loved one, unemployment, health issues, loss of a relationship, or financial or legal problems

Protective factors, sometimes referred to as resilience factors, are those things that provide protection from psychological problems following trauma. Some factors are things you can change (such as level of social support), and some factors are things you cannot change (such as age):

- Being part of a support group

- Relying on family or friends

- Absence or low levels of shame, guilt, or embarrassment related to the event

- Being naturally optimistic

- The ability to maintain a sense of humor

- Being older and having more life experiences

- Successful experience dealing with past difficult life events

- Effective coping strategies

Maintenance factors are those characteristics, attributes, and behaviors that maintain psychological distress following trauma. In essence, these are the things that keep you stuck in the trauma instead of allowing you to heal. Many factors can maintain psychological distress, but there are some common ones:

- Drug or alcohol abuse (including some prescription and over-the-counter medications)

- Self-demeaning thoughts (*It was my fault, I will never get better* or *I'm damaged goods*)

- Withdrawal from family, friends, and other social supports (community and religious groups)

- Not seeking professional help (although not everyone needs to see a mental health professional)

- Anger, resentment, and depression

The next exercise helps you identify the risk, protective, and maintenance factors in your life.

EXERCISE: My Factors—The Good and the Bad

As you work through this exercise, think about any personal factors that played a role in your adjustment following a trauma, whether these factors are positive or negative. Pay close attention to any personal factors that promote negative emotions and behaviors, particularly anything that can be changed. Record these factors as risk or maintenance factors in the space provided. Consider ways in which you can minimize their influence on you, and record how you can reduce their impact. Likewise identify any protective factors, which promote positive emotions or resilience, and consider and record some ways in which you can develop or strengthen them. Note that our previous list of possible risk, protective, and maintenance factors is by no means comprehensive. You may be able to think of other factors that have played a role in your own response to trauma. Write in your journal if you need additional space.

Risk factors:

1. _____

Explain how this factor puts you at risk. _____

How can you reduce its impact? _____

2. _____

Explain how this factor puts you at risk. _____

How can you reduce its impact? _____

3. _____

Explain how this factor puts you at risk. _____

How can you reduce its impact? _____

4. _____

Explain how this factor puts you at risk. _____

How can you reduce its impact? _____

5. _____

Explain how this factor puts you at risk. _____

How can you reduce its impact? _____

Maintenance factors:

1. _____

Explain how this factor maintains your symptoms. _____

How can you reduce its impact? _____

2. _____

Explain how this factor maintains your symptoms. _____

How can you reduce its impact? _____

3. _____

Explain how this factor maintains your symptoms. _____

How can you reduce its impact? _____

4. _____

Explain how this factor maintains your symptoms. _____

How can you reduce its impact? _____

5. _____

Explain how this factor maintains your symptoms. _____

How can you reduce its impact? _____

Protective factors:

1. _____

Explain how this factor helps you. _____

How can you maximize its impact? _____

2. _____

Explain how this factor helps you. _____

How can you maximize its impact? _____

3. _____

Explain how this factor helps you. _____

How can you maximize its impact? _____

4. _____

Explain how this factor helps you. _____

How can you maximize its impact? _____

5. _____

Explain how this factor helps you. _____

How can you maximize its impact? _____

Hopefully you now have a clear idea of the roles that various risk, protective, and maintenance factors have played in your life. Some of these factors can help you and others can keep you stuck in the past and make it more difficult to fully heal. Understanding this may help to protect you from the ill effects of traumas in the future. Our request is that you spend time every day finding ways to increase those factors that promote strength while eliminating or reducing those that keep you pinned down. An example of the former is to develop new friendships and expand your social network. An example of the latter is to reduce or eliminate your use of alcohol or drugs as a way to cope with your emotions.

Trauma Recovery

You may have already picked up on an important point implied earlier in this chapter. If up to 75 percent of people have been exposed to a traumatic event at some point in their life, and only 8 percent or so develop PTSD, most people either have little negative impact following trauma or have some post-trauma difficulties from which they recover over time. The truth is that the vast majority of people who suffer a trauma do not develop PTSD, although many may have some PTSD symptoms. And although most people will have some problems adjusting to a traumatic event, things will return to normal for them over time, usually within weeks or months. This is in part due to the strength of certain protective and maintenance factors in their lives. It is also a testament to the strength and resilience of human beings.

One only has to watch the evening news to see the death and destruction that people face every day. As psychologists, we are privileged to see the flip side—an incredible sense of perseverance, fortitude, and hope that permeates the human spirit. As you read this book, you will learn more about this flip side. And in addition to learning about why and how people recover from trauma, you will gain an appreciation for the ways that people can grow and become stronger following trauma. You will learn about posttraumatic growth and how to promote this growth in your own life as a response to the trauma or traumas you have suffered.

CHAPTER 2

How Trauma Affects Your Thinking

Consider for a moment the aftermath of an earthquake. We have all seen photographs or videos of earthquakes, and you may even have lived through one. Your own trauma was a psychological earthquake. Traumas have a magnitude just as earthquakes do. Some are barely felt, and others are so strong that little can withstand their effects. Furthermore, a city's roads, buildings, power lines, and sewers may be built to standards that allow them to withstand all but the strongest earthquakes, whereas some may be so weak that even a minor earthquake can bring everything crashing down. Similarly, your own reaction to trauma will depend on certain factors.

Looking at your basic beliefs as structures and the traumatic events in your life as earthquakes is a useful way to consider how trauma affects your own thinking. Imagine that your thoughts are like a city's infrastructure. You have an interconnected system of core beliefs that you hold about yourself, the world you live in, the people around you, your past, and your future. Some psychologists have called this system of core beliefs the *assumptive world*, since it reflects what you assume to be true in everyday life. Your own system of core beliefs is unique to you. These beliefs may seem obvious to you, and they serve you well. They make the world seem predictable, and if the world is predictable, you then know how to prepare for it, respond to it, or to control it (or at least you think you can). Like the infrastructure of a city—which provides shelter, water, travel, and power—your beliefs provide the basis for virtually everything you understand and do. And just as the city comes to a halt when its infrastructure is damaged, so it is with your brain in the aftermath of trauma: without it functioning the way it should, you come to a halt.

The Way It Feels When Trauma Hits

What does it feel like when a traumatic event functions like an earthquake? One thing many people say is that they "can't believe it happened," and they struggle for long periods of time to come to terms with the fact that it did. They know the fact to be true, but some part of them resists the difficult reality of what has happened. Each morning you may wake up with what feels like a new realization—it really happened. The old system of beliefs is still operating as if things were the way they were before the trauma. A mother whose child has died still thinks she will see him in his bedroom when she walks by, that he will return home from school, or that he will call on the weekend as he has done for years. She knows this is impossible, but it seems more impossible that her child is dead. The reality of life has always been, and therefore was always assumed to be, that the child lives. Furthermore, her assumption was always that her child would outlive her, and though she recognizes that parents sometimes outlive their children, it happens rarely. A further assumption might be that when children die first, it is always someone else's child. The often-reported experience of reliving the trauma appears to be an attempt to incorporate the fact of the trauma into the understanding someone has about life and how the world is supposed to be. This reliving of trauma can happen in dreams, in sudden flashbacks during the day, or in rumination about the traumatic events.

Another thing that happens to people when their core beliefs, or basic assumptions, are violated is that they are left wondering what to believe now. They feel that the world has suddenly become a strange place and that they need to develop a new understanding to account for what has happened. Again, there is a part of you that may say, "I know this sort of thing happens. I just didn't think it would ever happen to me!" The way life is going is unanticipated, odd, and difficult to navigate. Life no longer makes sense. For each of us, core beliefs help us to understand and predict events in life and therefore guide our plans and responses. If these beliefs no longer seem to function well because of the damage done to them by trauma, you can feel that you don't know what to do next or how to respond to an environment that now seems unpredictable and strange. In some ways, life appears to be what you knew, but that appearance, you know, is misleading. Things are different now.

As a survivor of trauma, you also may feel that this new world is a world you don't wish to be in. You don't want to understand it, because that would mean you are accepting something you would rather deny is true. So you wish to lodge a protest against this world that has changed and that has betrayed a system of beliefs you always held as true. After traumatic events, it is common for people to be angry for long periods of time. They are angry not only about what has happened but also about being forced into a position where they need to rethink how the world works, how life is going, and even who they are. These are very difficult tasks that they would prefer to avoid, and they long for the way that things used to be.

Trauma can change not only your environment but also your sense of who you are as a person. Just as we each use our system of core beliefs to understand our environment or other people, we also use it to understand ourselves and to anticipate what we are likely to do in various situations. Traumatic events often confront us with a need to respond, and we may be surprised by what we see in our own responses. Furthermore, trauma brings about other difficult circumstances that we need to respond to, and we may be surprised by our ability, or inability, to cope with them. So your beliefs about what kind of person you are may need a reevaluation as you take note of your own behavior during and after a trauma.

A trauma reveals important aspects of yourself and what kind of world you live in, and you may need to reconsider your future goals in light of these realizations. Perhaps certain goals that you had for yourself before the trauma are now gone, or perhaps these goals no longer seem to have as much meaning as they once did. Given what trauma has taught you, you may no longer believe that you can attain the goals that you had previously set. Or perhaps before the trauma you paid little attention to goals, but you now see a need for goals. Your future may need a closer examination than you have ever given it.

How Traumatic Events Affect You

How much you are struggling with the kinds of issues described above depends on your risk factors, your protective factors, and your maintenance factors (discussed in chapter 1). Your risk factors include the magnitude of the trauma and any weak spots in your core beliefs. Your protective factors include strong core beliefs and any help you might have in being able to strengthen them further. Maintenance of distress may occur when you do not have ways of revising your beliefs and feel stuck in the sense of disbelief or when you avoid thinking through what has happened. Your psychological infrastructure has been damaged in the aftermath of trauma, and you must develop a way to manage your situation so that you can function again.

One thing that makes it difficult to get a city functioning after an earthquake is aftershocks. Aftershocks can bring down already weakened structures and frighten the population so that it's difficult to get on with the process of recovery. People become wary, as they have no idea when an aftershock may occur. They are on edge and try to protect themselves from further danger. It is hard to know if you're really safe. Trauma survivors of all kinds also find themselves in this situation of feeling unsafe. A cancer survivor fears recurrence. A victim of crime stays on guard against another criminal attack. A person who is bereaved worries that another loved one will die. A soldier awaits the next ambush. The feeling that you are no longer safe in the world is a common post-trauma experience. It makes it difficult to think that life will ever be normal and that you can relax.

A major part of the problem is that trauma can affect your body as well as your mind, so you feel unsafe in both places. We are all built with an internal alarm mechanism that warns us of danger. This same self-protective mechanism that keeps us on guard against threat can cause us to worry. You may have the sense that if you stop worrying about the possible danger, you will be more likely to be victimized by it. Even if you understand that this is not really the case, the idea can be so compelling that you do not dare give up your vigilance. This is what psychologists call *intrusive rumination*. These are thoughts about the trauma and the strange world encountered in the aftermath of trauma. These thoughts come out of nowhere and seem impossible to control. They are typical early reactions to traumatic events although they may continue for months or even years. The more traumatic the event has been for you, the more likely you are to have these intrusive thoughts. This next exercise will help you assess the impact of the trauma on your thinking. The first part looks at how the trauma affected your thinking right after the event. The second part looks at the impact of trauma on your thinking now. The questions in the exercise are from Cann et al. (2011).

EXERCISE: A Self-Assessment of Intrusive Rumination

Immediate impact of trauma on thinking: Try to recall your thought processes immediately after the traumatic event—even if the event happened some time ago—and respond to each statement according to how you were feeling at the time. Circle the number underneath each statement that corresponds to how often, if at all, you had this experience during the weeks immediately after the event.

1. *I thought about the event when I did not mean to.*

0	1	2	3
Not at all	Rarely	Sometimes	Often

2. *Thoughts about the event came to mind, and I could not stop thinking about them.*

0	1	2	3
Not at all	Rarely	Sometimes	Often

3. *Thoughts about the event distracted me or kept me from being able to concentrate.*

0	1	2	3
Not at all	Rarely	Sometimes	Often

4. *I could not keep images or thoughts about the event from entering my mind.*

0	1	2	3
Not at all	Rarely	Sometimes	Often

5. *Thoughts, memories, or images of the event came to mind even when I did not want them to.*

0	1	2	3
Not at all	Rarely	Sometimes	Often

6. *Thoughts about the event caused me to relive my experience.*

0	1	2	3
Not at all	Rarely	Sometimes	Often

7. *Reminders of the event brought back thoughts about my experience.*

0	1	2	3
Not at all	Rarely	Sometimes	Often

8. *I found myself automatically thinking about what had happened.*

0	1	2	3
Not at all	Rarely	Sometimes	Often

9. *Other things kept leading me to think about my experience.*

0	1	2	3
Not at all	Rarely	Sometimes	Often

10. *I tried not to think about the event but could not keep the thoughts from my mind.*

0	1	2	3
Not at all	Rarely	Sometimes	Often

Current impact of trauma on thinking: Now circle the number below each statement that corresponds to how often, if at all, you had the experience described during the past two weeks.

11. *I thought about the event when I did not mean to.*

0	1	2	3
Not at all	Rarely	Sometimes	Often

12. *Thoughts about the event came to mind, and I could not stop thinking about them.*

0	1	2	3
Not at all	Rarely	Sometimes	Often

13. *Thoughts about the event distracted me or kept me from being able to concentrate.*

0	1	2	3
Not at all	Rarely	Sometimes	Often

14. *I could not keep images or thoughts about the event from entering my mind.*

0	1	2	3
Not at all	Rarely	Sometimes	Often

15. *Thoughts, memories, or images of the event came to mind even when I did not want them to.*

0	1	2	3
Not at all	Rarely	Sometimes	Often

16. *Thoughts about the event caused me to relive my experience.*

0	1	2	3
Not at all	Rarely	Sometimes	Often

17. *Reminders of the event brought back thoughts about my experience.*

0	1	2	3
Not at all	Rarely	Sometimes	Often

18. *I found myself automatically thinking about what had happened.*

0	1	2	3
Not at all	Rarely	Sometimes	Often

19. *Other things kept leading me to think about my experience.*

0	1	2	3
Not at all	Rarely	Sometimes	Often

20. *I tried not to think about the event but could not keep the thoughts from my mind.*

0	1	2	3
Not at all	Rarely	Sometimes	Often

Scoring: Add up the numbers circled for statements 1 to 10 to get your immediate impact score. Use this scale to determine the immediate negative impact of the event on you.

A score of 0–10:   No impact: this event was not traumatic. (Exceptions would be if the aftermath was too chaotic to clearly recall or if thinking was too difficult.)

A score of 11–15:   Minimal impact: this event may have been stressful but not likely traumatic. (Exceptions would be if the aftermath was too chaotic to clearly recall or if thinking was too difficult.)

A score of 16–20:   Significant impact: this event has elements of trauma.

A score of 21–30:   Major impact: this event was likely to be traumatic.

Add up the numbers circled for statements 11 to 20 for your current impact score. Use this scale to determine the current negative impact of the event on you.

A score of 0–10:   This event is not currently producing traumatic responses.

A score of 11–15:   This event is producing minimally stressful responses.

A score of 16–20:   This event is producing traumatic stress responses.

A score of 21–30:   This event is producing significant traumatic stress.

What You Have Found Out About Your Intrusive Thinking Then

So what have you discovered about what your thinking was like immediately after the traumatic event? You may not recall spending much time thinking about the traumatic event. Alternatively, it may be that you find it hard to think clearly about the immediate aftermath of the trauma, which is especially common for people if it was a chaotic time. There are situations where people are turning to survival, emotionally and/or physically, and they find themselves numb or preoccupied with other critical matters. This can happen in combat and at funerals. Therefore a low score could indicate that the event was traumatic for you, even if you do not specifically recall your thought patterns at that time. In such cases, there may be a delay in the development of disturbing thoughts about a traumatic event. Higher impact scores are common when a traumatic event can be immediately acknowledged.

What You Have Found Out About Your Intrusive Thinking Now

Now consider your tendency to ruminate now. This score on your self-assessment indicates the degree to which your thinking processes may have changed or remained the same since the event. If your score is lower than it was for the first ten questions of this assessment, you may have been able to bring your thinking into line with your existing belief system. Or it's possible you may be working on changing or developing your core beliefs. After a traumatic experience, people sometimes deliberately and intentionally spend time thinking about what has happened. This thinking process is sometimes called *deliberate rumination* or *reflective rumination*, which feels more constructive and under your control. This next exercise will help you assess the degree to which you are involved in core belief change or development. The first part looks at how much you were engaged in reflective thinking after the traumatic event. The second part looks at how much you are engaged in reflective thinking now. The questions in the exercise are from Cann et al. (2011).

EXERCISE: A Self-Assessment of Deliberate or Reflective Rumination

Reflective rumination since the traumatic event: Circle the number underneath each statement that corresponds to the degree to which you have in the past deliberately spent time thinking about these issues.

1. *I thought about whether I could find meaning from my experience.*

0	1	2	3
Not at all	Rarely	Sometimes	Often

2. *I thought about whether changes in my life have come from dealing with my experience.*

0	1	2	3
Not at all	Rarely	Sometimes	Often

35

3. *I forced myself to think about my feelings about my experience.*

0	1	2	3
Not at all	Rarely	Sometimes	Often

4. *I thought about whether I have learned anything as a result of my experience.*

0	1	2	3
Not at all	Rarely	Sometimes	Often

5. *I thought about whether the experience has changed my beliefs about the world.*

0	1	2	3
Not at all	Rarely	Sometimes	Often

6. *I thought about what the experience might mean for my future.*

0	1	2	3
Not at all	Rarely	Sometimes	Often

7. *I thought about whether my relationships with others have changed following my experience.*

0	1	2	3
Not at all	Rarely	Sometimes	Often

8. *I forced myself to deal with my feelings about the event.*

0	1	2	3
Not at all	Rarely	Sometimes	Often

9. *I deliberately thought about how the event had affected me.*

0	1	2	3
Not at all	Rarely	Sometimes	Often

10. *I thought about the event and tried to understand what happened.*

0	1	2	3
Not at all	Rarely	Sometimes	Often

Current reflective rumination: Now circle the number underneath each statement that corresponds to the degree to which you currently deliberately spend time thinking about these issues.

11. *I think about whether I can find meaning from my experience.*

0	1	2	3
Not at all	Rarely	Sometimes	Often

12. *I think about whether changes in my life have come from dealing with my experience.*

0	1	2	3
Not at all	Rarely	Sometimes	Often

13. *I force myself to think about my feelings about my experience.*

0	1	2	3
Not at all	Rarely	Sometimes	Often

14. *I think about whether I have learned anything as a result of my experience.*

0	1	2	3
Not at all	Rarely	Sometimes	Often

15. *I think about whether the experience has changed my beliefs about the world.*

0	1	2	3
Not at all	Rarely	Sometimes	Often

16. *I think about what the experience might mean for my future.*

0	1	2	3
Not at all	Rarely	Sometimes	Often

17. *I think about whether my relationships with others have changed following my experience.*

0	1	2	3
Not at all	Rarely	Sometimes	Often

18. *I force myself to deal with my feelings about the event.*

0	1	2	3
Not at all	Rarely	Sometimes	Often

19. *I deliberately think about how the event has affected me.*

0	1	2	3
Not at all	Rarely	Sometimes	Often

20. *I think about the event and try to understand what happened.*

0	1	2	3
Not at all	Rarely	Sometimes	Often

Scoring: Add up the numbers circled for statements 1 through 10. This score represents the degree to which you have engaged in reflective rumination in the past.

A score of 0–10: You have given little serious thought to the event.

A score of 11–15: You have given minimal thought to this event.

A score of 16–20: You have given significant thought to this event.

A score of 21–30 You have devoted a great deal of time and energy reflecting on the event and its aftermath.

Now add up the numbers circled for statements 11 to 20 to get the score for how much you currently engage in reflective rumination.

A score of 0–10: You are giving little serious thought to the event.

A score of 11–15: You are giving minimal thought to this event.

A score of 16–20: You are giving significant thought to this event.

A score of 21–30 You are devoting a great deal of time and energy reflecting on the event and its aftermath.

What You Have Found Out About Your Reflective Thinking

The reflective type of thinking that you considered in this self-assessment has been shown in our research to be directly related to the development of posttraumatic growth.

Reflective Thinking Then But Little Now

If you found that you have engaged in this reflective thinking in the past but are not doing so now, you might have essentially completed a process that has led to growth and change. Or perhaps as you engaged in reflective thinking, you tried to understand the experience of trauma but did not find any clarity in your understanding, and so you have deliberately stopped thinking this way. If that's the case, we hope that you will find this book to be a useful way to restart this process with more positive results.

Little Reflective Thinking

If you haven't ever engaged in reflective thinking about your trauma, we hope this book will help start this process for you. The fact that you are reading this book shows that you are ready to engage in this process, and we will help lead you through it.

Much Reflective Thinking

If your score indicated that you are currently engaging in a great deal of reflective thinking, you are in the midst of a process that can produce growth and change. We hope that this book will help you further this experience.

Reflective Thinking and Rebuilding

Deliberate rumination or reflective thinking allows trauma survivors to constructively approach developing a new belief system in the aftermath of trauma. When you move from intrusive rumination to deliberate rumination, you have a sense that you are more in control of what is going on in your mind. You are moving from the shock of confronting the destruction of your beliefs—or perhaps the startling recognition that you need to give more serious thought to how to live your life—to a place where you can build a new system of understanding that can survive this trauma and others in the future. Our earthquake metaphor can help in understanding this process.

In the aftermath of an earthquake, aspects of the infrastructure are typically destroyed to the extent that these aspects were weak in the first place or were facing the brunt of the trauma. Other aspects of the infrastructure may survive relatively unscathed, because they were more resilient. Perhaps they had been built in anticipation of the stress that an earthquake may cause. Likewise, you may have been vulnerable to trauma, or you may have been more resilient because your system of core beliefs included the possibilities of trauma and ways to successfully cope with it.

In the aftermath of an earthquake, it's important to get the city up and running again, but it's also important to take time to rebuild the city to be more resilient to future potential earthquakes and similar disasters. Similarly, as a trauma survivor, you may have needed to respond quickly, so you could continue living, and yet you also need to consider how to live successfully in the future. The latter comes with time, reflection, and hard work.

Accepting Help

In the short term, help may be needed from the outside to keep the city going and to rebuild. When the infrastructure has been shattered, the city is incapable of providing entirely for itself. Other agencies and individuals need to support the city with what is usually provided by the infrastructure—power, sanitation, medical supplies, food, water, and other basic needs. For trauma survivors, the situation is similar. In the immediate aftermath of trauma, it's hard to function normally, and finding support is necessary. Other people may provide not only assistance in getting through the day but also, in terms of your core belief system, a sense of hope, possibility, and something to think about. This allows you to continue to navigate the world that is now so strange.

Building a Resilient System

In the long term, the city needs to rebuild. This rebuilding should make the city more resilient so that it can withstand future tremors as well as larger disasters that now appear to be possible. Likewise, as a trauma survivor, you need to rebuild your system of core beliefs so that this internal system is resilient. This rebuilt system must incorporate the reality of what has happened and the possibility of future traumas, ways to cope with those traumas, and how to live life in spite of the uncertainty of when new traumas may occur or what they will be like.

The city must have stronger building codes in order to create a more resilient infrastructure. The trauma survivor must have better core beliefs, so the assumptive world fits better with the real world that may be encountered while allowing for a successful life within this world. The city rebuilt will be an improved version. The person with a new understanding of how to survive and thrive will be improved as well. Posttraumatic growth is the process the trauma survivor goes through to attain this new level of strength and resilience.

Where You Stand in the Process

You may now be in one of many phases of this process of posttraumatic growth. You may be in the immediate aftermath of trauma, in a state of disbelief, wondering what happened to your life. You may be trying to apply your old system of core beliefs to a situation that has radically changed, and you may now find this system to be inadequate. You may have experienced trauma some time ago and are already in the process of recovery. You are thinking about what your system of core beliefs needs to be and how to arrive at a system that works for you. Or you may have already done substantial work in developing a new way to understand your world, your future, and yourself and have a greater sense of confidence that you will be able to cope with future traumas. The self-assessments in this chapter have already helped to clarify where you are in this process of posttraumatic growth.

Now that you have an idea about how much your thinking process is either in a state of intrusion or reflection, you can assess what you may be thinking about. What aspects of your core beliefs, or assumptions about the world, may be undergoing reconstruction? This next exercise focuses on which of your core beliefs are in the process of reexamination or perhaps are undergoing serious reconsideration for the first time in your life. The questions in the exercise are from Cann et al. (2009).

EXERCISE: A Self-Assessment of the Challenge to Your Core Beliefs

Please reflect upon your traumatic event. Then for each statement, circle the number that corresponds to the extent to which the event led you to seriously examine a core belief.

1. *Because of the event, I have seriously examined the degree to which I believe things that happen to people are fair.*

0	1	2	3	4	5
not at all	to a very small degree	to a small degree	to a moderate degree	to a great degree	to a very great degree

2. *Because of the event, I have seriously examined the degree to which I believe things that happen to people are controllable.*

0	1	2	3	4	5
not at all	to a very small degree	to a small degree	to a moderate degree	to a great degree	to a very great degree

3. *Because of the event, I have seriously examined my assumptions concerning why other people think and behave the way they do.*

0	1	2	3	4	5
not at all	to a very small degree	to a small degree	to a moderate degree	to a great degree	to a very great degree

4. *Because of the event, I have seriously examined my beliefs about my relationships with other people.*

0	1	2	3	4	5
not at all	to a very small degree	to a small degree	to a moderate degree	to a great degree	to a very great degree

5. *Because of the event, I have seriously examined my beliefs about my own abilities, strengths, and weaknesses.*

0	1	2	3	4	5
not at all	to a very small degree	to a small degree	to a moder- ate degree	to a great degree	to a very great degree

6. *Because of the event, I have seriously examined my beliefs about my expectations for my future.*

0	1	2	3	4	5
not at all	to a very small degree	to a small degree	to a moder- ate degree	to a great degree	to a very great degree

7. *Because of the event, I have seriously examined my beliefs about the meaning of my life.*

0	1	2	3	4	5
not at all	to a very small degree	to a small degree	to a moder- ate degree	to a great degree	to a very great degree

8. *Because of the event, I have seriously examined my spiritual or religious beliefs.*

0	1	2	3	4	5
not at all	to a very small degree	to a small degree	to a moder- ate degree	to a great degree	to a very great degree

9. *Because of the event, I have seriously examined my beliefs about my own value or worth as a person.*

0	1	2	3	4	5
not at all	to a very small degree	to a small degree	to a moder- ate degree	to a great degree	to a very great degree

Scoring: Here is how you can determine the degree to which you have experienced a challenge to your core beliefs.

Primary score: Add up the numbers you circled for items 1 to 9.

0–10 You have little core belief disruption.

11–24 You have some core belief disruption.

25–45 You have substantial core belief disruption.

Secondary score: Look for the core beliefs that you have been seriously examining at the level of a 4 or 5. How many are there, and what are they?

_____

Core Belief Disruption and Growth

The previous assessment looked at how much you've been examining your core beliefs in the aftermath of trauma. There may be other particular beliefs that you have been reconsidering besides the nine core beliefs referred to here, but these nine are the general beliefs that tend to be shaken by the earthquake of trauma. They involve beliefs about yourself, the future, other people, and the way the world works.

It is important to consider both primary and secondary scores. A high score clearly indicates that you are reexamining your core beliefs, which can lead to posttraumatic growth. You may have a low primary score, indicating little core belief disruption but still have one or two beliefs on which you scored high. This indicates significant core belief disruption in a particular area. If you have any core beliefs that you have been seriously examining to a great degree or to a very great degree, you are likely in a process of reflection that can lead to posttraumatic growth.

Your Reconstruction Process

Reconstructing your belief system in the aftermath of trauma may be a difficult task. It may take months or, for some people, even years. This is because these beliefs are fundamental to who you are and they are put to use in almost all situations in life. To feel that life is understandable and that you know how to approach it, it's important to really check in with your core beliefs. We will return to considering these core beliefs in succeeding chapters, as you develop new perspectives on how trauma has changed you, the meaning of your life, and the story of your life.

Which of your core beliefs is challenged may depend largely on the circumstances. For example, a situation where you were disappointed in how you behaved or you feel guilty about your actions may make you question your belief about your value or worth as a person. This was the case for one man we know who was unable to save a friend from drowning. His friend fell overboard after having a seizure, and the man felt that he should have been able to prevent his friend's death, even though the incident had happened in the dark early hours of the morning, and the friend had fallen into murky water. Despite his best efforts, the man could not locate his friend. Following the incident, he came to question his ability to handle an emergency and to exert all the effort necessary to help another person. Merely being reassured by others was not enough to decrease his guilt, and he had to reassess his capabilities in the aftermath of this death.

On the other hand, if you went through a trauma where someone close to you betrayed you, you may need to reexamine your core belief about your relationships with other people. Marital infidelity is an example of a betrayal that often causes people to reexamine their core beliefs in this area.

Redefining Trauma

You may be surprised to read that marital infidelity could be traumatic, as it does not involve being confronted with physical threat or death. However, we consider many events to be *potentially traumatic events* because of their possible effects on the core belief system. The challenging of these beliefs—or the need to develop a clear system of beliefs to make sense of the event or to make sense of how to live life going forward—is what constitutes trauma for many people. Trauma is in the eye of the traumatized. We have found that what is usually the most difficult part of these events is a core belief system that is not up to the task of understanding what has happened or how to go on with real confidence. One man we knew was being treated with life-threatening cancer. Rich said to him, "I imagine this may be the hardest thing you have been through." The man said, "Actually, not. My divorce was much harder for me. That rocked my world." By that, he meant that his sense of his own value, his relationships, and his future were all called into question. His cancer, on the other hand, did not challenge his core beliefs. He was not surprised by this illness, because he had a family history of cancer.

Posttraumatic Growth as a Route to Resilience

Posttraumatic growth is the reconstruction of your belief system into a new system that did not even exist in any substantial form in the past. With this process comes a more resilient person, a person more capable of managing the traumas of the future. This is not unlike seeing a city rebuilt to higher standards through new understandings of how earthquakes and other potential disasters can affect its structures.

In the next chapter, you will learn how to confront the challenges to your core beliefs and begin to find a firm basis for living a satisfying life in the aftermath of your trauma. The disruption to core beliefs is emotionally upsetting; it creates anxiety, anger, and confusion. You must have a way of dealing with these emotional aspects of core belief disruption, so you can think yourself through to a new set of core beliefs and develop confidence in your own ability to manage your emotions and thoughts. You will learn some skills that will allow you to engage in the process of posttraumatic growth, as you construct new core beliefs you can count on.

CHAPTER 3

Processing Trauma and Its Aftermath

Managing the aftermath of a traumatic event can be difficult. The average person is flooded with different emotions, struggling to make sense of what happened and trying to find ways to make things "normal" again. Some people have support systems in place, which they can rely on for strength and comfort. Others have few to no resources to fall back on. Regardless of which group you fall into, this chapter offers some techniques and tools you can use to minimize the effects of difficult emotions that can be distressing or overwhelming. Learning to manage these emotions is an important step toward posttraumatic growth.

In addition to having strong emotions, many people battle unwanted and intrusive thoughts post-trauma. This is a normal and expected part of the healing process, as your mind tries to make sense of what happens to you after a tragedy. However, it's possible to get stuck, so you can't move past your thoughts. Through reflective thinking, you can turn these intrusive thoughts into a new story about what happened to you. As the author of your future, you can take control of your direction and explore new possibilities that may have been hidden for years. In the following pages, we will show you how.

Trauma and Emotions

In the days, weeks, months, and even years following a traumatic event, many trauma survivors struggle with a variety of strong and powerful emotions. Some people experience sadness and grief whereas others struggle with intense anxiety. Depending on the type of trauma, anger and rage may be the biggest emotional hurdles to clear. Outwardly directed emotions like anger are seen mostly in those who have suffered a very personal and intimate violation, such as a rape or an assault, or who have been harmed through the intentional action of another (this could include being injured by a drunk driver). And then there is guilt, or blaming yourself for what has happened.

People experience these emotions in different ways. Take anxiety, for example. Anxiety comes in many forms and goes by many names, such as worry, stress, nervousness, panic, or jitteriness. Just knowing how to label your anxious feelings may seem impossible, but the label is not so important. What's important is being able to recognize that what you're experiencing is anxiety, for then you can deal with it. It's also important to understand that everyone experiences various types and degrees of anxiety. So how do you recognize it? Some anxious people are worriers. They constantly think about what has gone wrong, is going wrong, or will go wrong. Others carry anxiety in their bodies. They carry around a constant tension in their shoulders or have this sinking feeling in the pit of their stomach. And some people, out of nowhere, experience these warm rushes throughout their whole body, which turns into fast breathing, sweating, dizziness, and shakiness.

Sadness is easier to identify. At some point, each and every one of us has had a period in which we were down, depressed, blue, or just felt plain blah. Sadness is a part of life. After trauma, though, sadness may become a daily part of your existence. You may struggle just to get out of bed in the morning, or you may avoid spending time with loved ones. Things you enjoyed in the past are no longer of interest to you. And it takes all your energy to do even the most basic things. For many trauma survivors, the driving force behind sadness is grief. This is especially true for those who are struggling because of the death of a spouse, parent, or child. Or your grief could be related to the loss of a job or intimate relationship. Basically, grief is the powerful emotional response we all experience when we lose something of value to us.

Anger has often been labeled as depression turned outward or toward someone else. As psychologists, we appreciate the simplicity of this view. However, we also understand that it's not so simple. Anger is a complex emotion. It's powerful and can lead to a variety of physical, emotional, relationship, and even legal problems. And if not controlled early in the aftermath of trauma, it can limit your ability to recover and grow from the traumatic event.

Guilt is also a complex emotion. Guilt is what you feel when you believe, whether you are right or wrong in your belief, that you have violated some personal moral standard. For example, a soldier who kills a female enemy on the battlefield may experience grief because of his actions. Even though he was trained to shoot the enemy, he still has a difficult time accepting the fact that he killed a woman. It goes against his beliefs about what's right and wrong. As another example, a mother whose child survived a terrible school bus crash feels guilty for being happy when other mothers were not so lucky.

As you can see, there are a number of emotions that can overwhelm a person following trauma. We refer to them as *negative emotions* not because they are bad in and of themselves but because they are painful and difficult feelings, and having them can make it hard to get through the day and move toward growth. And these are just a few of the feelings you may experience. At times, it may seem like you are drowning in your own feelings. You may feel frustrated that the traumatic event happened so long ago yet you are still struggling. Whether you are in the immediate days following the traumatic event or have suffered repeated traumas over your lifetime or are faced with continuing difficulties, there are ways you can better manage the negative emotions you're struggling with on a day-to-day basis. With five decades of combined experience and our work with thousands of people, we know how difficult this process can be. But we also know how resilient people are. We are constantly in awe of the incredible spirit and strength of the average person.

You can learn to manage your emotions. The exercises in this chapter are resources that you can use at any time and in a variety of situations. As you go through this process of growth, you will likely find it useful to frequently refer back to them. You may even find them useful in managing the day-to-day struggles we all face.

First we want you to take a few minutes to identify the different negative emotions that you may be experiencing related to your trauma. The goal is not to focus on what's wrong but to identify which feelings you may need to target.

EXERCISE: Name and Understand Your Feelings

The following lists of negative feelings include some that you may be experiencing. Circle the feelings that most seem to fit with your experience. Each list of feelings starts with a general feeling and follows with variations. You would circle the word *angry* if this matches your experience, but you may also want to circle another word or words to more closely describe the feeling you have, such as *enraged*, *furious*, or *outraged*. Circle whatever term or terms best describe your feelings.

Next, take a few minutes and think about which of these feelings are your most common feelings. What are your top three feelings? In other words, which three feelings cause you the most distress? Place a check mark next to those feelings.

FEARFUL	FRUSTRATED	ANGRY	DISGUSTED	APATHETIC
frightened	displeased	mad	tired of	stoic
apprehensive	disappointed	enraged	sick of	passive
hysterical	thwarted	aggravated	appalled	bored
afraid	defeated	outraged	disliking	cold
shuddering	aggravated	incensed	hating	unmoved
shivering	dismayed	infuriated	displeased	detached
terrified	upset	smoldering	outraged	distant
panicked	annoyed	indignant	nauseated	unemotional
timid	agitated	hot under the collar	horrified	indifferent
horrified	irritated		repulsed	numb
having the creeps	exasperated	livid		uncaring
		sore		removed
alarmed		irate		uninterested
dreading		furious		withdrawn
scared		pissed off		

GUILTY	TIRED	CONFUSED	SAD	STRESSED
ashamed	fatigued	baffled	bitter	troubled
embarrassed	overworked	bewildered	melancholy	distressed
remorseful	drained	ambivalent	heartbroken	upset
regretful	beat	dazed	depressed	on edge
humiliated	wiped out	hesitant	despairing	anxious
sorry	wasted	confounded	somber	cranky
hesitant	depleted	befuddled	pessimistic	distraught
shy	exhausted	lost	sorrowful	frazzled
bashful	finished	mystified	discouraged	irritable
distraught	lethargic	bemused	gloomy	anxious
	spent	perplexed	hopeless	nervous
	worn out	puzzled	unhappy	overwhelmed
		torn	down	restless
			low	unsettled
			blue	

Now look again at the three feelings that you feel most often, and use the space provided to reflect on two things. First say why you think these three feelings dominate the way you feel. Then try to describe how these three feelings affect your emotional and physical health. You can do this by simply writing down whatever comes to mind.

_____

_____

_____

_____

_____

_____

_____

_____

_____

The main goal of this exercise was to help you to identify the different feelings you experienced, or are still experiencing, after your trauma. Putting your different feelings into words can be helpful. You can benefit from this exercise even if you tend to use other words to describe how you feel. When you talk about your trauma with friends, family, a spiritual leader, or a therapist, you may want to see how some new feeling words fit into your discussions. And if you are not at a point where you can talk to others, strengthening your feeling vocabulary will help you better identify and process whatever you are feeling.

A secondary goal was to help you consider why your feelings may have so much power over you and what kind of impact they have on your overall well-being. In reality, we spend little time thinking about why we feel the way we do, and we move through life as if feelings are facts. The truth is that we have control over our feelings.

Taking Control of Your Emotions

Now that you've identified which distressing emotions you're experiencing, we'll teach you some new ways to manage them. In the following pages, we describe several effective techniques for managing strong emotions. These techniques are based on psychological research, and we have used them successfully with countless people. We know they work. However, they will work only if you practice them. Try to keep an open mind, and avoid automatically dismissing the techniques as too easy, too difficult, or too "psychological."

Take a Deep Breath

When you've been stressed, someone has probably told you to…you guessed it… breathe. There is no easier, cheaper, or more effective way to manage negative emotions than proper breathing. And it's not difficult to learn. We all have to breathe. Unfortunately, most of us do it wrong. The majority of people are chest breathers. This means that using your chest muscles instead of your diaphragm or stomach muscles to breathe. The easiest way to see how you breathe is to place one hand on your chest and the other on your stomach. Breathe normally. If you notice your hand on your chest moving up and down, then you are a chest breather. If the one on your stomach moves more, then you are a diaphragm breather. If you are a diaphragm breather, congratulations! If not, here's what you can do to change that.

Learning to use your diaphragm when breathing helps maintain balance within the *fight-or-flight system*, the delicate biological process that prepares us all for threats to our safety (fight or run) and returns us to normal when the threat is gone. The fight-or-flight system is generally set at a higher throttle in trauma survivors than everyone else, which makes it difficult to manage negative emotions and calm down. Deep breathing can help you lower that throttle and bring you back down to baseline. This in turn helps you manage negative emotions like anxiety, stress, anger, fear, and frustration.

EXERCISE: Diaphragmatic Breathing

Look around and find a quiet and comfortable place where you won't be disturbed. You'll need to be able to use this space for ten or fifteen minutes. It could be in your office with the door closed, at home in your bedroom, or outside away from distractions. Either lie flat or comfortably recline with your back and neck supported. Place your right hand on your chest and your left hand on your stomach. Slowly inhale through your nose. Hold your breath for a count of one and then slowly let the air effortlessly leave your body. As you breathe, make sure the hand on your chest stays still while the hand on your stomach rises and falls with each breath. Now as you breathe, visualize a balloon in your stomach. Each time you take a breath in through your nose, the balloon inflates. Each time you allow it to leave your body, the balloon deflates. Repeat this process for ten to fifteen minutes. And remember to make sure the hand on your chest stays still while the hand on your stomach goes up and down.

Practice this type of breathing for just a few minutes at least twice a day for two weeks to get good at it. You may want to practice in the morning before your day starts and in the evening before you turn in for bed. If you practice regularly, you'll be better able to use this technique when you need it to help you calm down.

You can also begin using this technique as situations arise throughout the day. For example, if you find yourself becoming nervous before making a trip to the store, take a few minutes to calm your fight-or-flight system before you leave the house. It will make the drive much easier. If your anxiety peaks once you pull into the parking lot, practice breathing in your car before going into the store.

Spend a few minutes writing and reflecting on this technique. Is it helpful? If so, why? If not, why not? Are there barriers to using it in your daily life? If so, what can you do to overcome those barriers?

_____

_____

_____

_____

_____

_____

_____

Relax with Progressive Muscle Relaxation

When stressed or frustrated, you've probably also had someone tell you to just relax. For the most part, it's good advice (though it can be hard to take if the person telling you to relax is being a bit condescending). The problem, of course, is that you may want to relax, but it feels like your mind and body are not cooperating. A relaxation technique called *progressive muscle relaxation* is an effective way to manage stress, anxiety, anger, and sadness.

EXERCISE: Progressive Muscle Relaxation

Find a quiet place where you can sit comfortably. You'll need to have this space to yourself for ten to fifteen minutes. As you sit comfortably with your feet on the floor and back straight, take a deep breath through your nose and exhale through your mouth. Do this for one or two minutes. Now shift your attention to your left foot. Slowly tense your foot by curling your toes under and squeezing tightly. Hold this tension for five seconds and then relax your foot. Do it again. Curl your toes under, hold for five seconds, and release. Notice the difference in how your foot feels as you tense and relax it. Now do the same thing for your right foot. Curl, hold, and release. And repeat. Now do the same thing for your calves, thighs, buttocks, back, shoulders, arms, face and forehead. Tense each part of your body, hold for five seconds, and release. Notice how your body feels in each of these tense and relaxed positions. Do this cycle twice for each body part.

Progressive muscle relaxation is another easy, inexpensive, and effective way to relieve stress, anxiety, anger, and a variety of other negative emotions that make relaxing difficult. Just as with deep breathing, muscle relaxation counters the fight-or-flight response to stress. And if you practice the technique twice a day, you will become a pro in no time and will be better able to use it when you need it. For example, you can use this technique at work after a difficult meeting, before a tough exam at school, or after an argument with a loved one.

Spend a few minutes writing and reflecting on this technique. Is it helpful? If so, why? If not, why not? Are there barriers to using it in your daily life? If so, what can you do to overcome those barriers?

_____

_____

_____

_____

_____

_____

_____

_____

_____

_____

_____

Imagery

Using imagery or visualization is another great way to keep the fight-or-flight system in balance. It's also a great way to resist negative thoughts that fuel sadness, grief, and guilt. Imagery allows you to temporarily remove yourself mentally and emotionally from your negative thoughts or chaotic and stressful surroundings. In essence, it acts as a positive distraction from your distress as it calms your mind and body. Below is an imagery exercise you can practice daily and use whenever stressful situations arise, to give yourself a break and a chance to manage your emotions. Read through it a few times first, so you are familiar with the flow of the exercise. Once you've got it, go ahead and start using it.

EXERCISE: Imagery

Find a quiet place where you can sit in a chair comfortably. You'll need to have this space to yourself for ten to fifteen minutes. As you sit comfortably with your feet on the floor and back straight, take a deep breath through your nose and exhale through your mouth. Do this for one or two minutes. You can close your eyes at any point. Allow the vision of a peaceful, safe, and comfortable place to enter your mind. It can be a place you've been to before or somewhere you've always wanted to go. It can even be a place that exists only in your mind. Once you can visualize this place, take some time to look around it. Pay close attention to the details of where you are. Spend thirty seconds noticing the colors that surround you. What colors do you see? How vivid are they? Spend thirty seconds noticing the different shapes in your place. Are there a lot of straight edges or curves? Take note of the temperature. Is it hot, cold, or just right? What sounds do you hear? Are there any smells you recognize? Spend as much time as you like noticing the surroundings in your place. When you are ready, slowly open your eyes and let your vision adjust to the light in the room. Notice how you feel once you have finished the exercise.

Using imagery is a great way to briefly leave the harsh reality that trauma leaves in its wake. It's not denial but rather a break from self-criticism and self-doubt, shame and guilt, and remorse. It's a preview of what can be or a memory of how things once were. When you find yourself consumed with negative thoughts, overcome with worry and fear, or unable to calm your mind and body, imagery can come to your rescue.

Spend a few minutes writing and reflecting on this technique. Is it helpful? If so, why? If not, why not? Are there barriers to using it in your daily life? If so, what can you do to overcome those barriers?

_____

_____

_____

_____

_____

_____

_____

_____

_____

_____

Check Your Thoughts

The Greek philosopher Epictetus is credited with the statement, "It's not what happens to you but how you react to it that matters." As psychologists, we agree but with one slight adjustment. We prefer to say, "It's not what happens to you, but how you _think about what happens to you_ that matters." More to come about thoughts soon…

Humans are far from perfect. We make mistakes all the time. This is especially true when it comes to our thoughts. In general, we are all prone to misinterpreting things that happen to us in life. This is not unique to trauma survivors. For example, a husband might think his spouse is cheating on him when she says she wants to spend the evening with her girlfriend once a week. In reality, she just wants to spend time with her friend. For trauma survivors, there is a greater tendency to perceive things in a negative light.

A plumber fixing a leaky faucet may be seen as a potential rapist by a woman who was sexually assaulted. Or the combat-weary soldier may think a bag of trash on the side of the road is a makeshift bomb.

These misinterpretations and misperceptions pop into the trauma survivor's head without warning, which can make you feel helpless over your thoughts. This helplessness leads to greater anxiety, sadness, anger, guilt, and many other negative emotions. But you are not helpless. In fact, you can control these thoughts and learn to replace them with more realistic and helpful ones.

You may already associate having certain thoughts and feelings together in response to certain situations. A form of psychotherapy called cognitive behavioral therapy (CBT) teaches that thoughts and feelings go hand in hand—that if you are thinking a certain way, it will make you feel a certain way, and vice versa. The following CBT exercise is designed to help you do three things. First it teaches you to recognize your *automatic thoughts*, thoughts that come in response to a situation or a triggering event. This is the first step in controlling automatic thoughts that fuel your negative emotions. Second, it allows you to test the reality of your thoughts. Much of the time automatic thoughts that fuel negative emotions have little basis in reality. You can test them and see that they are not true by identifying the evidence for and against your automatic thoughts. And last, through this exercise, you can find alternative, more realistic thoughts and views to replace the ones that contribute to your negative emotions. These alternative thoughts tend to lead to a more positive or neutral outlook about your situation.

EXERCISE: Keeping a Thought Record

Think of a recent situation or event that triggered an unwanted emotion. Fill in the blanks after reading the example.

1. What was the situation? Describe where you were and what you were doing.

    Example: *I was sitting in traffic on my way home after work. I saw this older couple talking and laughing with each other in the car next to me.*

    _____

    _____

2.   What was your emotion or feeling at the time? How strong was it?

Example: *I was feeling sad. On a scale of 1 to 10, it would have been an 8.*

_____

3.   What was your thinking at the time? What did you think automatically in response to the situation?

Example: *I will never be that happy with anyone ever again. Once David left, I lost my only chance for growing old with someone I loved.*

_____

_____

4.   What was the evidence supporting what you were thinking?

Example: *Some people only fall in love once, and the older you get the more difficult it is to meet people.*

_____

_____

5.   What was the evidence against what you were thinking?

Example: *I was in love with someone else before David, so there's no reason I couldn't fall in love with someone again.*

I have many friends and family who I love and they love me.

I will feel loved and love others for a long time.

_____

_____

_____

_____

6. What could you have thought instead in this situation? What is an alternative thought that would be more positive or neutral?

    Example: *I fell in love before, so I can fall in love again.*

    _____

    _____

    The goal of this exercise was simple. It was to help you identify, challenge, and replace automatic negative thoughts that lead to unwanted feelings that are hard to manage. If you practice this exercise regularly in response to situations that trigger negative thoughts, it will help you be less critical of yourself, feel less defeated or fearful, and set aside some of your shame or guilt. It's not offered to pretend that life isn't hard or that your struggles aren't real. It's a way to help you gain a different perspective—a perspective that will help you with the process of healing and recovery, a perspective that will get you on the road to growth.

    Spend a few minutes writing and reflecting on this exercise. Was it helpful? If so, why? If not, why not? Are there barriers to using this exercise in your daily life? If so, what can you do to overcome those barriers?

    _____

    _____

    _____

    _____

    _____

    _____

    _____

    _____

As you can see, the techniques we describe in this section are relatively simple. But though simple to use, they can be a powerful help in managing your emotions. As we said before, these techniques will work only if you practice them, so please do.

Taking Control of Intrusive Thoughts

Negative emotions are not the only unwelcomed consequences of trauma. Recurrent and intrusive thoughts plague many people after a traumatic event. Intrusive thoughts are unpleasant involuntary thoughts, ideas, and images. These unwanted intruders are a prominent and common symptom of the formal diagnosis of post-traumatic stress disorder. They are similar to the negative automatic thoughts discussed earlier. The main difference is that intrusive thoughts tend to be trauma focused. These thoughts replay portions of the traumatic event or events and are very distressing. You may feel helpless and unable to stop them, which further fuels negative emotions and reduces your ability to recover from the traumatic event. For example, when you have trouble controlling these reactions, you might start telling yourself that *I'm out of control* or asking yourself, *What's wrong with me?* This kind of thinking makes things even worse.

To move down the path to growth, it's important to gain control of these unwelcomed thoughts. Again, the first step is to increase awareness. The following exercise helps you to identify intrusive thoughts, images, and ideas that you may have.

EXERCISE: Recording Intrusive Thoughts

Think of an intrusive thought that you had recently. Identify any triggers that may have preceded your intrusive thought. This may take some time, as it is often not very obvious. Next, write out what the intrusive thought, idea, or image was that followed the trigger. Then reflect on the meaning behind it and write down your thoughts. For example, what does it say about you, if anything? What does the thought have to do with your situation? Then list any ways you coped or managed the thought. Fill in the blanks with your own situation after reading the example.

Situation or trigger:

Example: *A strange man knocked on the door.*

Intrusive thought, idea, or image:

Example: *The image of the man who attacked me popped into my head. I kept replaying the moment he put his hand around my mouth and threw me to the ground.*

_____

_____

_____

Interpretation (or what the intrusive thought means to you):

Example: *Since I'm still having these images so frequently, I don't think I've been able to move forward and put the assault behind me. I have more healing to do. Some part of me still thinks that all men are dangerous and out to hurt me.*

_____

_____

_____

Coping strategy:

Example: *I didn't answer the door. Instead, I spent the next ten minutes practicing my deep breathing and imagery exercises. I also spent some time reflecting on what things I need to do to better handle what happened to me. Finally, I called my friend Becky, who has always been a source of support and compassion for me.*

_____

_____

_____

After completing this exercise, you should have a better appreciation for the types of intrusive thoughts that are unique to you.

_____

Identifying your intrusive thoughts is only the first step. Next you must turn your intrusive thoughts into a new story through a deliberate reflection on what happened to you.

Reflective Rumination

The next step in managing unwanted and unwelcomed intrusive thoughts may seem unusual. That's because we're asking you to do something that may seem directly opposite to what you've done in the past. We'd like you to spend some time thinking about your intrusive thoughts instead of pushing them out or ignoring them.

Most people's initial reaction when confronted with a distressing thought or image is to get away from it as quickly as possible. This makes sense, because why would you want to make yourself feel bad by purposefully thinking about something bad that happened? In reality, however, avoiding the distressing thoughts gives these thoughts strength and keeps them alive. It also allows the thoughts to take on a life of their own. By trying to understand these thoughts about what happened to you, you get the opportunity to challenge errors in your thinking about what happened. As humans, we are prone to have errors in our thinking, and most of the time the errors are not in our favor.

So how do you think about your thoughts? It's through the process of reflective rumination (introduced in chapter 2). Reflective rumination is simply the process of deliberately focusing on those things that you are saying to yourself. This will allow you to determine what makes sense and how to most logically think about your trauma and its aftermath. The best way to accomplish this is to set some time aside each day to do nothing but focus on your thoughts.

EXERCISE: Reflect on Your Thoughts

Create a twenty-minute block of time each day to reflect on your thoughts. When you create this time for yourself is completely up to you. It may be before work or after you get home, or any time of day when you are not distracted by the chaos of work or school or other responsibilities. It's also important to delay any intrusive thoughts you may have during the day until you can think about them during this time that you've set aside. If unwanted thoughts pop into your head while at work or while shopping, just remind yourself that you've set time aside to think about these things. You can even jot down a quick note as a reminder, but then quickly move on with your day. Make sure that the time and place you choose to reflect on your thoughts is as free from distractions as possible.

Here is how we would like you to deal with your thoughts. As the thoughts enter your mind, simply acknowledge them. Avoid any attempt to push them out, label them, or pass judgment on them. Notice any emotions that they bring up for you. Do these thoughts tend to be harsh or critical? Are they self-blaming in nature?

Notice the general content of the thoughts as well as any themes that may connect them. If you find that a thought is too distressing for you, move on to another one or come back to this exercise later. In this way, you are becoming a neutral observer of your own thoughts rather than having emotional reactions to them. This is a first step toward getting control over them. Strangely enough, in order to get control over your thoughts, you are now just letting them be what they are and noticing them. It's as if you were a scientist observing yourself, collecting the data on what your mind does.

Once you are comfortable allowing yourself the time to acknowledge and reflect on your thoughts, the next step is to check them for accuracy. Again, we are all prone to making errors in our thinking. We assume things to be true when in reality they are not. And in most cases, we tend to be hard on ourselves rather than give ourselves some slack. The reasons we do this vary, but it's often a by-product of how we grew up. As children, we do our best to make sense of the confusing world around us. Unfortunately, our experience is limited and we tend to draw incorrect conclusions about things. For example, if our parents get into an argument, we may think it's our fault, or if our teacher is in a bad mood and yells at the class for being too loud, we may think she is directing her anger at us and may label ourselves as bad. These early perceptions follow us into adulthood in many different forms. Therefore, as an adult, it's important to periodically check the correctness of your thinking.

EXERCISE: Questioning the Evidence

Use the space provided to log your intrusive thinking after you have had time to reflectively ruminate. For each thought, look for the evidence that supports it. Then look for the evidence that doesn't support the thought, or challenges it. Once you have completed the first two steps, see if you can come up with an alternative thought or statement that is more based in reality and probability. Do this for each of your intrusive thoughts to reveal the errors in your thinking and to come up with a more positive outlook. An example is provided.

Your intrusive thought	Evidence for the thought	Challenging the evidence	More realistic thought
Example: *It's my fault Marie was killed by the drunk driver.*	*I was driving the car that night.*	*The drunk driver is the one who crossed over into our lane. I didn't have a chance to react.*	*The drunk driver was responsible for her death. He chose to drink and drive. He passed out at the wheel and ran into us.*

It's our hope that with reflective rumination, you will be better able to identify errors in your thinking, particularly those errors that may be contributing to your distress and keeping you from seeing new possibilities.

We believe that how you think and what you say to yourself directly affects how you feel and how you behave. If your feelings and behaviors are fueled by negative errors, then your feelings and behaviors will be inconsistent with how you want to be. Unless corrected, this pattern will prevent you from opening new doors in your life and keep you stuck in the past. Once you unlock those doors, you will be confronted with many new possibilities for your future.

A Few Final Thoughts

As we mentioned earlier, the greatest paradox of posttraumatic growth is that out of loss, there can be growth—a new story of meaning and integrity and of a life that rewards you. This is the ultimate point of the book. Even in the face of unthinkable tragedy, possibilities for growth are waiting for you. Where you once were vulnerable, you can be strong and resilient. Everyone's story is different, but they all hold the possibility of growth.

The most important thing to remember is that your life after trauma is not fixed or static. It can change, and you have the ability to shape your future any way you like. This process is neither easy nor quick. It takes time, hard work, and the courage to rely on those around you with whom you find comfort and support. Those people in your life who understand what you've gone through and who appreciate the strength that already resides inside of you can be of greatest help.

Over the next few chapters, you will gain a better understanding of the various ways in which people tend to grow after trauma. And you'll learn various strategies for living a more meaningful life. You will also continue to rely on the strategies you have learned in this chapter and build on them. It's our hope that you are starting to realize that good can come from the bad and that all things are possible if you believe in and work toward a better life.

CHAPTER 4

The Varieties of Growth

In chapter 3, you learned more about some of the unwanted and troubling emotions and thoughts that can result from trauma. You also learned some new ways to manage your natural responses to trauma to reduce the impact of these symptoms and to gain control over them. But we want to help you do more than that. This book is also about the positive ways you can respond to traumatic events and grow from them. This chapter will go into this topic in greater detail and give you a chance to move in this positive direction.

This chapter will describe what posttraumatic growth looks like for many people and guide you through the process so that you can make the most of your opportunity to change the aftermath of your trauma into a time that you value rather than dread. We know that posttraumatic growth is not something that is easily or quickly experienced by most people; this is not to be discouraging but to emphasize that merely reading this workbook will be just the beginning of a process that takes time. We also believe that the information and exercises in this chapter can help you wherever you are in this process.

Getting Ready to Experience Posttraumatic Growth

Doing certain kinds of things can indicate that you're in a good position to experience posttraumatic growth. People who do these things are more likely to actively seek opportunities for growth. As you read through this list, ask yourself if you already are doing some of these things and if there are others that you could do as well. This list can provide you with an idea of what you can do differently to advance the process of growth.

I try to do things that I find personally enjoyable or engaging.

I do projects or work that I love.

The important activities in my life are often activities that involve the people I love.

I make sure to spend time with people who are dear to me.

I actively seek new ways in which to think about life, even if it means I've been wrong all along.

I ask people what they think about different social issues (on topics like politics, religion, culture, economics, lifestyles), so I can understand different points of view and develop my ability to think about life.

I choose new projects or activities based on whether they will help me develop my mind.

I consciously think about my connection to society and culture.

I set realistic goals for what I want to change in my situation or about myself.

I know how to make a realistic plan in order to make changes.

I ask for help when I try to make changes.

I know steps I can take to make changes in myself.

I know when it's time to change specific things about myself.

The fact that you are reading this workbook is an indicator that you are interested in personal growth. You are almost halfway through at this point, so you are persisting in this process. This is a very good sign. It means that you are already on the path to growing in spite of your trauma and suffering.

Posttraumatic Growth Takes Various Forms

What posttraumatic growth is like for you will be different from what it is like for others. There are different forms of posttraumatic growth and different combinations can happen within each individual. The kind of trauma you experienced, what you were like beforehand, and what you have been exposed to afterward all play a role in determining what form of growth you experience. As you learn more about what posttraumatic growth can look like, you will have an opportunity to move in specific directions much more deliberately than someone who is dealing with their life after trauma without the knowledge or guidance offered in this book.

You may recognize that you have already begun to experience some aspects of growth. You may already be experiencing growth in certain ways, and as you recognize the positive changes that are occurring, you can build on them. If you are not yet seeing growth, we want to give you an idea of what could happen for you in the future. It's hard to achieve what you cannot imagine. So be aware of these possibilities or imagine these things.

Our research has shown that there are five general types of posttraumatic growth that people report: personal strength, improved relationships with others, appreciation of life, new paths and possibilities, and spiritual change and a new understanding of life's meaning and purpose. We discovered these five forms of positive change as we interviewed people who were doing particularly well in the aftermath of trauma, listened to their stories, and later analyzed what we heard.

Personal Strength

Many survivors of trauma are surprised to discover their own internal strength. Most of us would never imagine being in a situation where we needed that kind of strength, but if we had imagined it, we might not think we could bear being in a car wreck, being the one diagnosed with cancer, or being the parent whose child has died. Although we all realize that it's possible for bad things to happen to us, it may seem that they are other people's life experiences, not yours. What's amazing is that when it does happen to you, you find a way to manage what you're going through, discovering a strength that you had never known or needed before.

Some trauma survivors do not think of themselves as special, despite their ability to survive. They might say to those who admire them or see them as a hero, "What else was I supposed to do? Give up and die?" But your strength as a survivor of trauma is something worth recognizing.

In struggling with a highly stressful event, you may realize that you can handle extremely difficult problems. The daily battle with post-trauma difficulties leads some people to develop a greater degree of self-reliance. They realize that they can face extreme situations successfully. Many people who have lived through traumatic life events have told us that after going through their difficulties, they felt that other troubles would seem trivial by comparison. They've told us that they discovered psychological resources that they never before realized they possessed. They were able to manage their emotional distress, solve problems, and make significant changes in their lives.

You might find yourself noticing some of these strengths in yourself. Just as necessity is the mother of invention, for many people, trauma may be the mother of strength. Whether this strength was there all along or developed in the aftermath of crisis is unclear. Regardless, many people who survive a crisis come to realize it.

Here is what Victor, a young man who battled cancer, told us. "I am stronger psychologically. I can handle any stress situation—struggle makes any stress situation something that can strengthen you." When asked specifically about what had produced this sense of personal strength, he said, "I have been through so many ups and downs with this. I have had to be sick and miserable for so long. I have lost so much time to this disease. I have come up against the thought of giving up, more than once. At some point, I just marveled at myself, *Hey Vic, you're still here!* It was hard to believe how much I could endure. It started to become like some crazy challenge, like 'Bring it on!' I know it sounds crazy, but I got to find out how much I can take, and it was a source of some pride."

Nobody would volunteer to experience a tragic event, but the lesson is clear. In your struggle to survive, to cope, and to prevail, you are given an opportunity to develop a strength you didn't know you had. The struggle can make you stronger, even as you experience the pain that goes along with the trauma.

Here are some statements from people who have noticed or developed personal strength as part of the growth experience. These statements are based on what people have told us about their growth after trauma, such as the death of a loved one or physical disability. See to what extent you would agree with them:

I am better able to accept the way things work out.

I have a greater feeling of self-reliance.

I know better that I can handle difficulties.

I discovered that I'm stronger than I thought I was.

These statements reflect personal strength. You need personal strength to cope successfully with trauma, and trauma may be a testing ground that reveals these strengths in you. For example, coping successfully requires the ability to accept things as they are. Many traumatic events cannot be changed. Being angry, resentful, or depressed about something that cannot be changed is a waste of time and energy. People who are able to absorb what is now the new fact of life and focus on dealing with their new reality will do better. They can also begin to appreciate themselves for having the ability to do this.

Here again we want to be sure that you do not misunderstand something crucial. Acceptance is not the same as giving up. Accepting something that may be difficult to accept does not mean that you can't change other things in your situation. For example, a soldier who has suffered wounds that resulted in amputations must accept that his limbs are gone, but he does not have to accept that he will no longer be physically active. He may find the strength to focus on how to live with prosthetic limbs rather than give up on life.

Acceptance about everything related to your trauma also does not have to come all at once. You may be able to accept some things more easily than others. For example, a widow once told Rich that she could accept her husband's death after a long bout with cancer, as he was now at peace rather than in pain. But it was harder for her to accept living alone, especially at night, where she felt most lonely without his company. It was also harder to accept that she would never again have in her life the kind of love that they had shared. Still, she was able to recognize that she had shown a great deal of personal strength during her husband's illness when he needed a lot of medical care. And after his death, she had kept many friends and been active with them despite her grief. She had been married almost fifty years and did not ever consider how she could live without her husband, but she found she was doing just that.

This brings us to a second kind of personal strength that you may recognize in surviving trauma: appreciating your ability to rely on yourself and to face hardship. Some parts of what you are going through you must do on your own. No one else is going to live your life for you. You have to live it, whatever it now may be. The ability to face up to this, and to see that you can live this new life using your own personal resources, can be a source of pride and comfort. Here are some questions that will help you appreciate your own personal strength and growth since your trauma (Tedeschi and Calhoun 1996).

EXERCISE: Recognizing Your Strength

Respond to each question in the space provided.

1. What have you done to cope that most clearly demonstrates the strength that has gotten you through this difficult time?

_____

_____

_____

_____

_____

2. What are some things that seemed difficult before the trauma that now seem relatively easy for you, given what you have gone through?

_____

_____

_____

_____

_____

3. What advice might you have for others who think that a situation similar to yours is too difficult to manage?

_____

_____

_____

_____

_____

What did you learn about yourself from completing this exercise? You may be stronger and more capable than you previously realized. Write about your experience in your journal.

_____

Improved Relationships with Others

An important part of the post-trauma experience is to find and accept concern from other people. While self-reliance is important, since no one can live out the aftermath of trauma for you, so is finding and accepting support. Accepting support brings you closer to others. You may find that your relationships become stronger and more intimate, in part, as a result of learning how kind and compassionate other people can be. Your relationships may improve with family members, friends, or even the general human family.

One couple we worked with was dealing with their son Charlie's drug addiction and eventual disability from the brain damage that it had caused. Charlie's mother described what Charlie's problems have done to her relationship with her husband. "I know that something like this might pull a lot of couples apart, but it has had the opposite effect with Glenn and me. I think we were kind of going our own ways before, focused on work and career aspirations, but now we've come together as Charlie's parents. We've had to make some tough decisions together, and Charlie is dependent on both of us to help him. And sometimes it is such a struggle that Glenn and I have to be able to tell when the other needs a break. We are much more of a team. We've also seen each other's pain in all of this, and we are much closer emotionally. I see a side of Glenn I never knew before, very tender and protective. And it makes me love him even more and show it too!"

See how your views of your post-trauma experience fit with the statements below.

I learned a great deal about how wonderful people are.

I more clearly see that I can count on people in times of trouble.

I have a greater sense of closeness with others.

I am more willing to express my emotions.

I receive more compassion for others.

I put more effort into my relationships.

I better accept that I need others.

You may notice two general themes in these statements about how relationships with others may change as a result of trauma. One is that your trauma has helped you see that you can count on others and accept their help. This is an aspect of growth because there is strength in being able to accept help. Men especially have often grown up with the idea that accepting help is a sign of weakness. Consequently, growth for many men involves the recognition that you can deal with difficulties more effectively if you seek help or accept it when offered. While men are prone to this idea that they must be weak if they need help, they are also raised to believe that teamwork is important. Thinking of accepting help as part of a team may make it easier for men. At some point, all of us need other people, and the acceptance of our need for others is an important lesson that trauma teaches us. Learning to accept your own limitations and vulnerabilities may allow you to appreciate the help of others more.

The other theme is that you can gain a greater appreciation for other people and begin to put more effort into your relationships. You learn that there are others who care about you. And as your compassion grows and your recognition of your own imperfections and needs increases, you have a greater chance of growing closer to other people. This is not to say that in times of need everyone will respond as you wish. Some people may disappoint you. Many survivors of trauma have stories of how people whom they thought they could count on were insensitive or absent. But most often there are some surprises, where people whom you may not have even expected to notice or respond have been especially kind.

Here are some questions to help you enhance your relationships with others in the aftermath of trauma (Tedeschi and Calhoun 1996).

EXERCISE: Enhancing Your Relationships

Respond to each question in the space provided.

1. Were there people who pleasantly surprised you when you needed help after or during the traumatic or stressful situation? How can you show your appreciation?

    _____

    _____

    _____

    _____

    _____

2. Who are the people who could best understand what you have been going through? How could you communicate with them?

_____

_____

_____

_____

_____

3. What do you now understand about being a human being that you did not fully understand before you went through your difficulties? How can you put that understanding into action?

_____

_____

_____

_____

_____

What changes in your relationships with others have you noticed in the aftermath of your trauma? You may have felt nurtured by others, established new relationships, or found ways of being better connected to others. Write about your experience in your journal.

_____

Appreciation of Life

Perhaps one of the most common lessons learned from experiencing loss is that life has much to offer. You are left with a greater appreciation for what you have. You may discover that your priorities have shifted. Most frequently, it is the enduring and everyday areas of life that people come to appreciate the most. For survivors of trauma, each simple aspect of life may be a wonderful gift.

The loss or threat of loss forces many people to confront how precious life can be. This confrontation can lead to a radical change of priorities and to a greater understanding of what is truly important. For most people, this radical change does not occur without the shattering experience of major loss, or at least the threat of a major loss. It's like the old saying, "You never miss the water till the well runs dry." The struggle with trauma forces people to confront, evaluate, and change their priorities.

Consider the extent to which you agree with each of the following statements:

I changed my priorities about what is important in life.

I have a greater appreciation for the value of my own life.

I can better appreciate each day.

Traumas that threaten your life can make you appreciate the mere fact that you are alive. We often see survivors of floods, hurricanes, wildfires, and tornadoes speaking in front of their demolished homes. Many say, "We are so grateful to be alive. We can replace the stuff we lost but not each other." Some people talk about surviving a trauma as bonus time. Consider Malcolm, a young man who was badly wounded in a drive-by shooting: "I came this close to not being here. I've seen lots of people who got shot, but you know, I thought, *Who cares if I die? So what?* But when it really happened, I was so scared. I knew I wanted to live. Never knew I wanted it that bad. I really gotta take care of myself now. Take care of my life. I got another chance. I don't want to blow it."

This appreciation for life can show up in gratitude. It can lead people to offer prayers of thanks. It can lead people to slow down and savor their everyday lives. You may literally slow down to smell the roses, or pay careful attention to what your five senses bring to your experience. You may choose to eat slower and truly taste your food. You may take time to look around you. You may pay closer attention to the sensations in your own body.

Appreciation for life takes many forms. We have seen some people be more careful, take fewer risks, and then we have seen others who have done the opposite, and both types of people say they have learned to live in a way that makes the most of their life experience. Both are reporting a change in their perspectives and how they approach living in a way that expresses it.

An example of appreciating life by living it with more care is Luis, who lost his hand in an industrial accident. Here is what he said about how he has changed his approach to living.

"Of all people to have this happen, I couldn't believe it was me. Fifteen years at the plant—I had been the safety steward on my shift! Then this machine breaks and wham! It got me. So I figured I was useless now. Without a hand, I couldn't do this work. I was not going to be able to provide for my family. I was done. But the doctors started working with me to get me a new hand, a prosthesis. The doctors and their assistants spent a lot of time on me, and I started to think, *I can't give up, these people are working too hard for me to just give up on them, and myself.* And my family stuck by me. They didn't see me as useless. Lucky for me, the company, or the insurance, paid for things. If not for that, maybe I would have gone down the drain. But I started to think that there were a lot of good people working for me and that life was good—look what I had, all these people caring for me! I was also forced to slow down—I couldn't do my old routines. And doing stuff with one hand, man, it took forever to do things that are easy—easy with two, anyway. So that slowed me down. At first I was frustrated, but I had to learn to go with it, not be frustrated. So slowing down became something I started to do with everything, and it was like being deliberate about everything, noticing things. That is real different for me.

"Before, I couldn't wait to do stuff—I was very impatient and trying to get everything in, as much as possible. I would go out with my buddies and play basketball at night and stay out until midnight and then get up for work early. I always liked to do the stuff that was a thrill. I always seemed to want the adrenaline rush. Then, it all changed, and I changed with it. First, I resented it, losing the way I used to be. But now, I realize it's good. I talk to my kids. I am at home more. I am not impatient and irritable. It's because I have learned how lucky I am to have people who have stuck with me, even though I used to be so self-centered. I think I am a better man. My wife thinks so! I appreciate her more, too."

Here are some questions that will encourage you in appreciating your own life (Tedeschi and Calhoun 1996).

EXERCISE: Appreciating Your Life

Respond to each question in the space provided.

1. What have you lost or come close to losing as a result of your trauma that you didn't value enough before? Are there some things in your life now that you could demonstrate a greater appreciation for?

    _____

    _____

    _____

    _____

    _____

2. Do an experiment of slowly moving through a place familiar to you—in your house, your yard, your workplace, a public space, a natural area—and carefully take note of the smallest things. Look at things, listen to things, touch things, smell things, as if you were a child exploring them. What have you noticed in doing this?

    _____

    _____

    _____

    _____

    _____

3. Introduce a little extra time into certain activities of your day, so you can savor them. These could include eating, bathing, a chore, or your interactions with loved

ones, friends, or even people you hardly know, such as a store clerk. What have you noticed as you have done this?

_____

_____

_____

_____

_____

What have you noticed that you appreciate about yourself and your life in the aftermath of trauma? There may be things that were easier to overlook prior to the trauma. Answer this question in your journal.

_____

New Life Paths and Possibilities

Changes in your life path can be as great as a complete change in careers or as simple as increasing the degree to which you help out others who have experienced a variety of traumatic events. One outcome you may notice in yourself is that you hold more strongly to certain beliefs that guide your actions. These beliefs may reflect a new appreciation of life, and your priorities can change as you appreciate life more. Or it may be that you have new priorities or goals because the trauma has shut the door on old priorities and goals.

One young woman we worked with had been an athlete who was training for Olympic-level competition. Alice's whole life was focused on this goal. She became disabled after being in an auto accident and considered working toward the Paralympics. But during her time in rehabilitation, she became much more devoted to helping other patients who were struggling. Here is what she said about how this experience changed her priorities and goals. "After the accident, I was angry that my dreams had been dashed. I had been working toward my Olympic goals since I was ten. But I have always been determined, and so I figured I could still be a great athlete, but now a Paralympic athlete. So that was my mind-set. Not too different from what I had always been and wanted to be. I was still going to find a way to be me. Then a strange thing started to happen. While I was in rehab, I saw other people struggling to recover, and the kids especially. I wanted to help them and motivate them. I started paying more attention to them than to my own goals. And one day, I realized my goals had changed. I didn't really want to win medals anymore. I got more out of seeing other people succeed. Especially when they surprised themselves, I loved it! So this was my new goal. And you know, I feel much better about it. I feel more giving and less selfish. Before it was all about me. People admired me for my athletics, but now people love me for my generosity."

Notice that the change in Alice sneaked up on her. She didn't realize that the change was happening. We want you to take time to consider changes in yourself. Think about what may be becoming most satisfying for you, most important, and how these new beliefs could become the basis for new goals in your life. Consider the statements below to see to what degree you may be on the pathway to new possibilities for your life.

I developed new interests.

I established a new path for my life.

I am able to do better things with my life.

New opportunities are available which wouldn't have been otherwise.

I am more likely to try to change things that need changing.

Certainly the switch from previously held goals and life paths to new ones will involve some sense of loss. For many people, putting aside what has been important for many years is difficult. Old goals and paths provided a sense of meaning and purpose. They may have been a basis for a great deal of success in life. You can't expect to switch to a new life path without some struggle and grief. This is another example of how posttraumatic growth does not come without struggle and without confronting loss. Out of these losses, however, something even more important and useful to you may emerge. Just think of Alice, who gave up a lifelong goal of becoming an elite athlete when she found that providing help to others gave her more satisfaction, drew her closer to people, and perhaps could provide meaning long after athletic achievements were no longer possible.

Here are some questions that may encourage you to see new possibilities in your own life (Tedeschi and Calhoun 1996).

EXERCISE: Seeing New Possibilities

Respond to the questions in the space provided.

1. Are there some activities and interests that no longer seem as important to you now as they once were? Take a close look at why that may be and how you view these interests now versus before.

_____

_____

_____

_____

_____

2. What kinds of things do you wish you could do if you were not considering the practicalities involved?

_____

_____

_____

_____

3. Are there some small ways you can begin to integrate into your life the things you wish you could do?

_____

_____

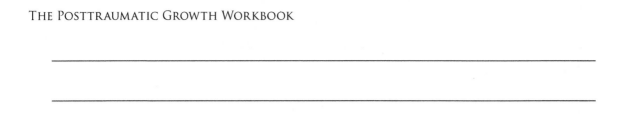

_____

_____

_____

What has become more important to you during your struggles? How can these things find a way into the life you are living and will live going forward? Answer these questions in your journal. You may notice that these changes were unplanned, surprising, and subtle. Try to turn them into more definite goals for yourself.

_____

Spiritual Change and a New Understanding of Life's Meaning and Purpose

As you struggle to make sense out of what has happened and as you wrestle with the trauma you have encountered, you may face the task of trying to fit what has happened into the beliefs you have held. And as you struggle and wrestle with what has happened, an increased sense of the importance of spiritual matters, or an understanding of how to live life well, may be a result. Because of the trauma, things about life that were previously upsetting may have become trivial in comparison. You may even have some impatience with others who remain focused on such issues, who don't have the perspective that trauma can bring. A new perspective may come easily to you, or if you are like most people, it will involve an intensive and even long struggle with the major questions about the purpose or meaning of your life.

When we talk about these new perspectives on how to live life well, you may think about your religious beliefs, your spiritual sense, or your philosophy of life. Many people find guidance in scriptures while others seek it in more secular teachings and ideas. Many people find their own truths not in the words of others but in a very personal way that seems to come from within. Consider the statements below that represent some ways that people can change spiritually, in the broadest sense of that term.

I have greater clarity about life's meaning.

I have a greater sense that I am part of the fabric of life.

I feel better able to face questions about life and death.

I have a deeper sense of connection with the world.

I have a better grasp of what life is all about.

The key is to seek your own truth for how to live life well. And if you haven't figured it out yet, this is less important than the fact that you are searching. In fact, trying to determine how to live your live well is more a process than a specific answer to a question. For example, if you are a Christian and have concluded that the answer to how to live well is to follow the teachings of Jesus Christ, you still have to figure out how to do that in this complicated world. Then you have to implement those teachings throughout your everyday life.

In some ways, trauma makes philosophers out of people. Many of us go through life not paying much attention to such questions as "What is the most important thing I can be doing with the time I have on this earth?" Or "Was I put here for a purpose?" Or "After I am gone, will my life have mattered?" Instead, most of us simply go through the daily routine and survive another day. Traumas force us to reconsider these questions or to consider them for the first time in a serious way.

One Vietnam War veteran described being shot down in a helicopter and the effect it has had on him ever since. In his description, we can see this aspect of growth: "The rotor blades were breaking apart. The fire was all around. We crashed and rolled on the side of a hill. I have never experienced a feeling like the one I had at that moment. The greatest experience of my life was occurring. The leaves on the trees were the deepest color green I had ever seen. In the encounter with the North Vietnamese troops, I wanted to capture them, not kill them. I did not want to deprive potential children of their fathers. I had to return fire to avoid being killed myself and to prevent their entry into our perimeter. I compare everything in my life to that experience. It is a question of whether or not I am being loyal to the experience. I simply know whether my actions and attitudes are in line with the experience of completion I experienced on that day in June."

One of the things that some people mention, as they describe what has changed in their deepest beliefs, is the idea of knowing things in a different way. As this veteran said, "I simply know."

Here is another example of this kind of knowing, described by a bereaved mother:

"And I realized before—well, you say you realize things, you read stuff and say, 'Yeah, that's right, like God first, and then your marriage, then your family and children.' And something like this happens, and it becomes more real to you—that priority and what's important. So you know it maybe intellectually before, but you realize it in a different way."

In dealing with your experience of trauma, you may already be involved in the process of addressing the big questions of how to live life well. Wherever you are in this process, here are some questions that may help you identify and use the principles that make sense to you (Tedeschi and Calhoun 1996).

EXERCISE: Finding Meaning and Purpose

1. What do you realize now that you never clearly realized before the trauma?

_____

_____

_____

_____

_____

2. What things did you think you knew before that you now know with greater conviction?

_____

_____

_____

_____

3. Do you have questions about how to live your life that are unanswered and perhaps even uncomfortable for you to consider? What are they?

_____

_____

_____

_____

_____

What do you understand to be the deeper lessons of your experience? You might consider how to put this hard-won wisdom into practice in a way that brings you greater satisfaction in living your life. Write your answers to this question in your journal.

_____

Some Concluding Words

The forms of growth we have discussed here are sometimes experienced as knowledge or wisdom achieved but are more often experienced as a work in progress. The fact that you are reading this workbook probably indicates that growth is still a work in progress for you. We think that people who see things this way are probably going to make the most of the difficulties of their traumatic experience. If you think you don't have things all figured out, you will continue to search and will find even more growth and change in the future. If you think you have found everything, you will stop searching.

We all wish to be comfortable, but getting uncomfortable has its set of own rewards. Therefore, this workbook is designed not to get you comfortable but to encourage you to stick with the discomforts you will experience on the path to posttraumatic growth. Of course, when people get too uncomfortable, they start to avoid things, and as we have mentioned before, avoidance is not the most useful way to deal with life after trauma. So we hope that you are finding enough comfort in this workbook to continue on the path to growth. The next few chapters will provide more information on how to engage in a process of searching that is fruitful and rewarding.

CHAPTER 5

Building Strength

Trauma can shatter a person's belief system. An unthinkable tragedy can upset your most strongly held beliefs about how the world is supposed to be. Your views about personal safety and the safety of loved ones may be turned upside down. Your beliefs about fairness may be crushed, so questions like *Why me?* become all-consuming. We've discussed how this is normal and common for many trauma survivors. Feeling vulnerable is also common in the aftermath of trauma. You may question your own personal strength, particularly your ability to handle what's happened. This chapter focuses on how it takes a great deal of strength to navigate trauma and its aftermath. The central paradox to this aspect of posttraumatic growth is that recognizing your own vulnerability is key to being strong after trauma. As you learn to appreciate your own strength, you will also see how it can provide resilience in the face of future misfortune.

Building Strength Takes Time

Many trauma survivors question why they have not bounced back within the days, months, or even years following a tragedy. For many, this questioning leads to negative and destructive feelings like shame, guilt, and despair. The reality is that everyone navigates the aftermath of trauma differently. There is no universal timeline for growth. It happens for some more quickly than for others. And we are not all that great at predicting who will respond more quickly.

What we can say with a considerable degree of confidence is that people tend to recognize their own personal strength only after some time has passed following the trauma. It is not immediate, but in most cases it does occur. Why does this take time? Trauma typically leaves people feeling weak and confused, and it takes time to get past these feelings. This is understandable. Until something happens that causes us to rethink our core beliefs about the world and ourselves, most of us move through life assuming that these beliefs will never be shaken. We possess varying degrees of confidence in ourselves, which have been created over years of winning many victories like graduating from school, finding a mate, or landing a job. When this confidence is shaken by the death of a loved one, sexual assault, or a near deadly car crash, we are knocked back on our heels. We begin to question those things that we thought we knew about ourselves. Thoughts such as *Maybe I'm not so tough after all* and *I am weak and helpless in this dangerous world* invade our thoughts.

However, this questioning of your strength should not be confused with weakness or your inability to overcome hardship. It should be viewed as a temporary diversion. You've been blindsided and hit hard. You've been knocked off your path, and you're temporarily dazed and confused. No, this is not permanent. It's part of the healing and growth process. This process is best seen in the story of a soldier Bret worked with while in Iraq:

"Before that stray rocket landed in our camp, and Eric was killed and I was injured, I thought I was invincible. I was such a good soldier. I was fast and strong. I pulled guys out of burning trucks and killed enemies who were within seconds of killing me and my buddies. For months after the incident, I felt so weak. I felt so helpless. It was the first time in my life that I felt vulnerable. I hated that feeling. My commander pulling me from missions didn't help. I just hung out in my room thinking about how useless I had become. It wasn't until my sergeant talked with me that things started to change. He shared with me how he experienced these same feelings after one of his soldiers was killed on his last deployment. He described the guilt he felt that he could not save this kid who he was responsible for. He eventually realized that dwelling on the loss of this one soldier put the other soldiers he was responsible for in danger. Instead of focusing on the death of one, he focused on saving the lives of the dozens he was in charge of. His sharing his experience made me realize that I was an important part of a team, and that my guys needed me out there. I had the experience to help keep them safe. Once my Sergeant put me back on missions, my confidence started to grow. The feelings of weakness eventually left. I became a better soldier and more connected to my guys."

This story highlights a few key points. First, the weakness and confusion following trauma are temporary. Second, talking with others can help you gain a different perspective and clarity. And third, overcoming negative ruminations by getting back on the horse and gaining new life experience leads to recovery and growth. Although this soldier's case is unique in its circumstances, it is not unique in its outcome. The story of being shaken and feeling defeated but eventually getting on the path to growth is common.

Here are some questions to help you assess your beliefs about safety before your trauma.

EXERCISE: Safety Before Trauma

Respond to the questions in the space provided.

1. Think back to the time before your traumatic experience (or first traumatic experience if you've suffered repeated traumas). How would you describe your views about your personal safety? How confident were you that you could keep yourself safe?

_____

_____

_____

_____

_____

_____

_____

Prior to the trauma, how would you rate your ability to keep yourself safe? Use a scale of 1 to 10, with 1 being not at all and 10 being completely. Circle one.

1   2   3   4   5   6   7   8   9   10

2. Prior to the trauma, how would you describe your ability to keep others safe?

_____

_____

_____

_____

_____

_____

_____

_____

Prior to the trauma, how would you rate your ability to keep others safe? Use a scale of 1 to 10, with 1 being not at all and 10 being completely. Circle one.

1   2   3   4   5   6   7   8   9   10

3. Before the trauma, what were your views about how safe the world was in general? Overall, was it a safe place? Was it filled with danger? What things made it safe or dangerous?

_____

_____

_____

_____

_____

_____

_____

_____

Prior to the trauma, how safe would you have rated the world? Use a scale of 1 to 10, with 1 being not at all and 10 being completely. Circle one.

1   2   3   4   5   6   7   8   9   10

4. Considering that we all feel weak at times, how would you describe the degree to which you saw yourself as weak prior to the trauma? At what times did you feel the weakest?

_____

_____

_____

_____

_____

_____

_____

Prior to the trauma, how would you have rated your overall level of weakness? Use a scale of 1 to 10, with 1 being not at all and 10 being completely. Circle one.

1   2   3   4   5   6   7   8   9   10

This exercise gives you a feel for your sense of safety and personal strength before you experienced the trauma. This is a baseline from which you can compare how you felt later.

_____

Following trauma, your sense of safety as well as your sense of personal strength may have changed. Here are some questions to help you explore any difference between then and now.

EXERCISE: Safety After Trauma

Respond to the questions in the space provided.

1. How would you describe your views about your personal safety now? How confident are you that you can keep yourself safe?

    _____

    _____

    _____

    _____

    _____

    _____

    _____

On a scale of 1 to 10, with 1 being not at all and 10 being completely, how would you rate your ability to keep yourself safe? Circle one.

   1   2   3   4   5   6   7   8   9   10

2. How would you now describe your ability to keep others safe?

    _____

    _____

_____

_____

_____

_____

_____

_____

On a scale of 1 to 10, with 1 being not at all and 10 being completely, how would you rate your ability to keep others safe? Circle one.

1   2   3   4   5   6   7   8   9   10

3. Describe your views now about how safe the world is in general. Do you feel it is a safe place? Is it filled with danger? What things make it safe or dangerous?

_____

_____

_____

_____

_____

_____

_____

_____

On a scale of 1 to 10, with 1 being not at all and 10 being completely, how safe do you rate the world now? Circle one.

1   2   3   4   5   6   7   8   9   10

4. Considering that we all feel weak at times, how would you describe the degree to which you see yourself as weak now? When do you feel the weakest?

_____

_____

_____

_____

_____

_____

_____

On a scale of 1 to 10, with 1 being not at all and 10 being completely, how would you rate your overall level of weakness now? Circle one.

1   2   3   4   5   6   7   8   9   10

These exercises together can help you assess if your beliefs about safety and your own personal strength have changed since the trauma. If your views of personal safety and your own strength have changed very little, it could be because you've already made significant gains since your trauma. If your views have changed a great deal, the trauma may be still relatively fresh and you are just beginning on the path to posttraumatic growth.

_____

Pay Attention to the Signs

How do you know if you are making progress toward recovery and growth? There are signs, but they can be easy to miss because they are often subtle. In fact, unless you deliberately spend time searching, it's unlikely you will notice them. And if you aren't seeing them, we ask you to trust us, for they are most certainly there.

What does strength look like? The short answer is that it depends on the person. Each of us comes to the table with different types and degrees of strength. It may be that you have greater courage in social situations. It could be that instead of withdrawing from the unfamiliar, you are more comfortable approaching strangers at a party or at work. Or it could be that you start to talk more freely with loved ones about the trauma.

A good way to recognize your various strengths is to look at how your life has changed, and is changing, in three core areas of life: family, work (or school or child-rearing), and social relationships. The next exercise will help you identify your personal strengths.

EXERCISE: Recognizing Your Strengths

Make a list of strengths you possess within your family, in your work, and in your relationships. Describe how you know that these are strengths and whether they existed before the trauma. If they existed before the trauma, describe how they have gotten stronger. If these strengths are new, describe how they developed. If you run out of space, use your journal to list and write about any additional strengths you possess. If you get stuck and can't recognize any of your own strengths, ask someone who knows you well.

Family strengths. List your strengths, as a spouse, parent, sibling, or child, within your family, and answer the questions that follow. Use the space provided after the example.

Example:

I have shared more intimate information about myself with my husband.

How do you know this is a strength? What's the evidence?

My husband commented to me that he's happy that I'm sharing more personal information about myself with him. He also told me he feels more connected to me emotionally.

Did this strength exist prior to the trauma, or is it new? If you've always had this strength, how has it changed? If it's new, how did it develop?

No. This did not exist prior to the trauma. I have always been very careful about what I tell my husband. I think I was afraid of scaring him off or that he would think I'm crazy. I'm pretty sure this new strength developed because I desperately needed someone to talk to, and he was willing to listen. I'm glad I took the risk.

Family strength 1: _____

How do you know this is a strength? What's the evidence? _____

_____

_____

Did this strength exist prior to the trauma, or is it new? If you've always had this strength, how has it changed? If it's new, how did it develop?

_____

_____

Family strength 2: _____

How do you know this is a strength? What's the evidence? _____

_____

_____

Did this strength exist prior to the trauma, or is it new? If you've always had this strength, how has it changed? If it's new, how did it develop?

_____

_____

Work strengths. Identify your work-related strengths and answer the questions that follow. Keep in mind that work is defined here in a broad sense, not just a nine-to-five job. Your work may be going to school or taking care of children and the home.

Work strength 1: _____

How do you know this is a strength? What's the evidence? _____

_____

_____

Did this strength exist prior to the trauma, or is it new? If you've always had this strength, how has it changed? If it's new, how did it develop?

_____

_____

Work strength 2: _____

How do you know this is a strength? What's the evidence? _____

_____

_____

Did this strength exist prior to the trauma, or is it new? If you've always had this strength, how has it changed? If it's new, how did it develop?

_____

_____

Relationship strengths. Identify your relationship-related strengths, such as relationships with friends, peers, or strangers, and answer the questions that follow. Add family and work relationships if you did not include them in the previous two exercises.

Relationship strength 1: _____

How do you know this is a strength? What's the evidence? _____

_____

_____

Did this strength exist prior to the trauma, or is it new? If you've always had this strength, how has it changed? If it's new, how did it develop?

_____

_____

Relationship strength 2: _____

How do you know this is a strength? What's the evidence? _____

_____

_____

Did this strength exist prior to the trauma, or is it new? If you've always had this strength, how has it changed? If it's new, how did it develop?

_____

_____

Additional strengths: Use the space below to identify any additional strengths you notice about yourself that do not fit into one of these three categories. For example, you may notice strength in your faith and spirituality or in your emotional and physical health.

Additional strength: _____

How do you know this is a strength? What's the evidence? _____

_____

_____

Did this strength exist prior to the trauma, or is it new? If you've always had this strength, how has it changed? If it's new, how did it develop?

_____

_____

Additional strength: _____

How do you know this is a strength? What's the evidence? _____

_____

_____

Did this strength exist prior to the trauma, or is it new? If you've always had this strength, how has it changed? If it's new, how did it develop?

_____

_____

We hope this exercise has helped you to better identify the various strengths you currently possess, particularly if these strengths are new. This is part of the growth process. It's important to continue this type of deliberate review and analysis of your life. This is the only way to truly appreciate your inner strength.

Coping Mechanisms: Using What Works

An important way to develop strength and resilience is to use healthy coping mechanisms. Coping mechanisms are defenses against stress and psychological discomfort. They can be used consciously or unconsciously and are often categorized into *adaptive*, or healthy, behaviors, and *maladaptive*, or harmful, behaviors.

Which type of coping behavior you tend to choose is largely based on your previous experiences: what you learned from your family as a child and what has and has not worked for you in the past. You may reject coping mechanisms that don't work for you; however, since many of these behaviors are deeply engrained and rooted in your childhood, you may keep using them even when they don't work. Here are some common coping mechanisms people use.

Negative coping mechanisms: criticize yourself/say negative things about yourself, use alcohol or drugs, avoid family or friends, act out aggressively/violently toward someone, overeat or not eat enough, keep your emotions bottled up, call in sick to work/school when you're not sick, shout, scream or yell at someone, throw something, drive fast, intentionally harm yourself (cutting), throw something, bite your fingernails, worry about things, criticize or blame others, smoke

Positive coping mechanisms: meditation, deep breathing/relaxation, humor/laughter, read a book/watch television, take a bath or shower, listen to music, pray or go to church, draw, paint, color, or write, talk with a family member or friend, work in the garden/yard, exercise, take a nap, go to a movie, engage in a hobby, scream into a pillow, cry

These two lists are by no means complete—there are thousands of different coping mechanisms that people use—but they give you an idea of the difference between positive and negative coping. It is also important to realize that going to extremes with a coping mechanism can sometimes make it unhealthy—for example, sleeping too much, or watching TV too much, or exercising too much. Be aware of when attempts to cope get in the way of other activities or interfere with your relationships. The next exercise will help you see which coping mechanisms you are already using and whether they are healthy or unhealthy.

EXERCISE: Your Coping Mechanisms

Create a list of the coping mechanisms you use to deal with stress or uncomfortable situations. If you tend to use any that we listed under positive and negative coping mechanisms, write them here, and add any others that you use. Place a check mark next to each coping mechanism that you list to indicate whether the way you are using it is positive or negative:

_____ positive _____ or negative _____

_____ positive _____ or negative _____

_____ positive _____ or negative _____

_____ positive _____ or negative _____

_____ positive _____ or negative _____

_____ positive _____ or negative _____

Now that you have a better idea about the coping mechanisms that you are already using, you're in a better position to decide if you want to make any changes. It's important for your posttraumatic growth to replace any negative coping mechanisms with positive ones.

The importance of positive coping mechanisms following trauma is that they allow you to manage the emotional and physical symptoms trauma causes. Without them, you would have no ability to fight off the ill effects of what's happened to you. It's a bit like the role of antibodies in fighting off infections. When you become infected with bacteria or a virus, your body mobilizes specific proteins (antibodies) that wage war against the foreign invader. The same is true psychologically. When you are confronted with the emotional and physical consequences of trauma, your mind can mobilize positive coping strategies to fight back.

However, if you have found that you tend to use a lot of negative coping mechanisms to cope with the trauma, it will make the process of growth much harder. If you are having a difficult time, and a lot of time has passed since your trauma, it could explain why the aftereffects are continuing to be so difficult for you. If your coping mechanisms are negative, we'd like you to make a pledge that you will try to replace them with positive coping mechanisms.

EXERCISE: Make a Pledge

I pledge to try my best to replace my most frequently used negative coping mechanisms with positive ones. I will do this by

_____

_____

_____

_____

The negative coping mechanisms I plan to stop using include

_____

_____

_____

_____

I pledge this on this date _____, _____.

Signed,

_____

In our work over the years with all types of clients, we've found that the simple act of making a pledge to yourself can have tremendous benefit.

There is one more important thing we need to point out about coping mechanisms: they can be helpful but only up to a point. Yes, they are helpful in fighting off the effects of trauma, but relying too heavily on them will keep you stuck and make achieving growth more difficult. That's why finding what works is important. Having a variety of coping mechanisms is usually best, especially since some may be more appropriate for certain circumstances than others.

Again, confronting the distressing aspects of your trauma is key to moving forward. A little avoidance can be useful in providing temporary relief from distress, but consistently avoiding confronting the trauma is not. Therefore, knowing when to confront trauma and how much to do it is critical. It's a lot like a dosing schedule for treating allergies. If exposed to very low doses of an allergen over time, a person can develop a tolerance to the allergen. As the tolerance to the allergen increases, eventually, the person no longer has a reaction to it.

Unfortunately, there is no perfect formula for determining how much confrontation is too much or not enough. It really depends on you. A good rule of thumb is to confront your distressing thoughts, feelings, and reminders of the traumatic event even though you may be upset and find yourself wanting to stop. But if you start to feel like you are losing control or becoming too overwhelmed, you can always pull back. Remember that the longer you confront your trauma, the easier it gets. Eventually, the trauma will have little to no emotional hold on you and will be replaced with a newfound meaning and purpose.

Asking for Help

We've talked about how there are many paradoxes associated with posttraumatic growth. For example, from loss can come tremendous gain; from vulnerability and weakness comes strength and resilience. Here's another: one of the primary ways of showing strength and resilience during periods of vulnerability is to ask for help.

Modern-day Western society is based on the idea that people should be independent and self-reliant. We are inundated with messages from television, movies, and newspaper and magazine articles about how we should "be strong" and "not rely on other people for our happiness." Independence and self-reliance are important. But taken to the extreme, they can be harmful to recovery and interfere with growth.

Asking for help is one of the most important ingredients in posttraumatic growth. Without assistance and support from others, you will be limited in what you can accomplish. Think about it. If you look back on your life and consider some of your most prized accomplishments, you will likely see how others helped you succeed. We do not live in isolation, and rarely do we accomplish anything without some level of assistance from others. But following trauma, people tend to withdraw from others and refuse to ask for help. This leads to continued despair and is a roadblock to posttraumatic growth.

The reasons people are hesitant in asking for help vary. Some say they are afraid of being rejected or are embarrassed and ashamed. Others don't want to be a burden, or they have internalized the idea of being independent and self-reliant to such a degree that they have never learned how to ask for help. It's also important to let go of your pride. It's common to try to maintain an attitude of being strong. You may want to have a reputation of being strong because society places so much value on being independent and self-reliant. But trying too hard to be or look strong for others also gives the impression that you have no needs, so others may not recognize how you are hurting. This leads you to feel lonely, isolated, and not understood. This is a particular problem for men, as society places an even higher expectation of stoicism and self-sufficiency on them, but it occurs in women as well. And if left unchecked, it will most surely keep you stuck in the past.

Remember, strength is necessary to navigate trauma and its aftermath, and it comes in many forms. At times, it may seem like you have little left in your reserves. The truth, however, is that strength lies deep inside you. It exists in your vulnerability and weakness. It resides in your ability to ask for help and seek support from those around you. It shows when you let down your guard and trust that others understand and care about you. As you proceed on the path of posttraumatic growth, it's important to keep these things in mind. Your inner strength is what has gotten you to this point, so far. Our hope is that you are able to unlock its full potential, so you will do more than just live. It's our hope that you will flourish.

CHAPTER 6

Compassion and Companionship

You need compassion and companionship for both recovery and growth after trauma. *Social support* is a term many professionals use when talking about this. It simply means having people help you get through the tough times, and a lot of books on trauma recovery will encourage you to get the social support you need. While we agree that social support is good in general, we believe it can be most helpful in the form of a particularly good companion on your journey after trauma. We call this kind of person an *expert companion*. In using this term, we don't mean to imply that this companion has to be a professional or have received any special kind of training. Rather, this companion is an expert at providing a sense of compassion and understanding for you in the aftermath of your traumatic experiences.

You may already be fortunate enough to have one or more such companions in your life. This chapter talks about how expert companions can help you grow after trauma. If you have no one in your life who fits this description, we will guide you toward finding someone. We will also talk about how you can become an expert companion to offer this kind of support to someone else in difficult circumstances. This may happen once you have made greater headway down the path to growth. Perhaps you have already found it happening to you.

On the Journey with an Expert Companion

What is it like to be with an expert companion? Most importantly, it is easy to just *be*. That is, an expert companion has no expectations for you to do things a certain way and instead allows you to be comfortable just being yourself. That might mean being your sad self at times, your angry self at other times, your frightened self at still other times. Whatever you are feeling, an expert companion is comfortable with you, so you do not need to change. We use the word "companion" to emphasize that this is a person who can stick with you on the journey through the tough times in trauma's aftermath. A companion goes with you, doesn't push you, and experiences much of what you experience along the way. A companion is someone who waits when you need a break and provides a helping hand when you slip. A companion stays by your side. A companion shares the experience and is interested in how you are doing. Your companion wants to listen to your description of the experience and tries to see it through your eyes. At the same time, the companion can offer a sense of perspective.

Expert Companions Stay Focused on Your Needs and Strength

In the aftermath of trauma, the journey is one that you, as the trauma survivor, are directing. You will need to chart the course of this journey, since it is personal to you. Expert companions are accepting of this fact and understand that their role is mostly passive, although there may be times when they are more active in providing assistance. They don't become frustrated with the pace, because they realize that this journey is harder for you than it is for them. They do not require a clear sense of the endpoint or of how much assistance you may need along the way. They are comfortable with this uncertainty while having faith in your ability to continue on this path to some unknown destination. But expert companions also have faith in your ability to do well. They understand that as a result of this journey, you will become someone more than you were. They understand that growth is a real possibility and encourage you toward it by pointing it out to you along the way.

Expert Companions Provide Guidance When It Is Useful

At a time in your life when you may feel less able to see things clearly, understand what is happening, or sense what direction to take, an expert companion can step in with some guidance. An expert companion points things out that you miss, especially about yourself and the progress you are making. An expert companion offers ideas about what might be happening without acting like a know-it-all. An expert companion remains respectful of you even when you have trouble respecting yourself.

Now, you may be thinking that you have never had a relationship like this, or you may be reminded of a special relationship. To get a sense of how important such a relationship can be, here are some questions to reflect on.

EXERCISE: Experiencing Expert Companionship

Answer the following questions in the space provided.

1. Think of a time when you felt most understood by another person. Who was it?

_____

2. What things did that person do or say that gave you the feeling of being understood?

_____.

_____.

_____.

_____.

_____.

3. Think of a time when you felt misunderstood by another person. Who was it?

_____

4. What did that person do or say that gave you this impression?

_____

_____

_____

_____

5. What could that person have done differently, which would have made you feel understood?

_____

_____

_____

_____

_____

Expert companions are compassionate and are sensitive to your needs. If you have had this kind of experience with someone in the past, it will be easier for you to recognize the sort of relationship that will be most helpful to you in your difficult circumstances.

_____

Being subjected to hurtful or disappointing relationships in the aftermath of traumas just makes everything harder. On the other hand, expert companionship is the best kind of relating in the aftermath of trauma. Expert companionship is especially helpful for posttraumatic growth.

How Expert Companions Help with Posttraumatic Growth

You have already learned a lot about how you can move toward growth in the aftermath of trauma. Much of this process involves experiencing strong emotions and dealing with thoughts that intrude on you and seemingly cannot be dismissed. The posttraumatic growth process also involves reflecting on important beliefs that have been challenged by what has happened to you and the building of new beliefs and a new vision for your future. Expert companionship can help you with all of this. Here is how this works.

Expert Companions Help with Emotions

After a traumatic event when you feel your most intense emotions, an expert companion can help you feel these feelings without shame. Knowing that your feelings are okay to express will allow you to say more about them and understand them more deeply. Simply being able to say what you are feeling is a relief. Exploring your feelings in more detail is even better for you. This is because the feelings you are having may feel foreign. You may never have felt things so deeply. An expert companion who allows conversations around these unusual feelings is essentially saying to you, "Anything you are feeling about this is okay with me, and I am not going to judge you or leave you because you feel a certain way."

Expert Companions Help with Intrusive Thoughts

When you experience intrusive thoughts about traumatic events and their aftermath, an expert companion can be someone to share these with, allowing them to be off-loaded, so to speak, and contained by this other person. It can feel good when someone else knows what you have been thinking and accepts these thoughts without judging you. It provides you with a sense that you are not alone with these disturbing ideas. One client recently said to Rich, "When I leave your office, I think about leaving all this here, and I can come back to it later."

Expert Companions Help You Sort Out What to Believe

When you examine your core beliefs or try to figure out what to believe, an expert companion can be a sounding board for you. It's helpful to be able to say what you think out loud. An expert companion listens to your thoughts as you try to figure out what to believe. While helping you get your thoughts organized, the expert companion never criticizes what you say or tells you what is right or wrong to believe. An expert companion may offer you a different perspective but in a way that does not imply that you have to accept it.

Finding What Works for You

No one is going to be a perfect expert companion. The key is to find someone who is good for you. In fact, different people need different versions of this kind of companionship. You might need different things from your expert companion at different times.

You may not be used to indicating what your needs are. You also may not understand what it is exactly that you would like to have in this relationship. Here is a list of many of the things that people need at various times from an expert companion. You can use it to figure out what you need and how to express your needs to someone else.

EXERCISE: What You Need from an Expert Companion

Check off the things that you need from someone right now.

- ☐ Someone who will listen to how I am feeling without judging me.

- ☐ Someone who will let me know if I am thinking in a way that makes sense or not.

- ☐ Someone who will encourage me.

- ☐ Someone who will let me cry.

- ☐ Someone who will let me be angry.

- ☐ Someone who is okay with me being confused.

- ☐ Someone who can be okay with just not talking.

- ☐ Someone who has some experience with what I am going through.

- ☐ Someone who has a sense of humor.

- ☐ Someone who lets me know what he or she is thinking.

- ☐ Someone who does not push ideas on me.

- ☐ Someone who does not try to tell me what to do.

- ☐ Someone who will take me seriously.

- ☐ Someone who will let me take my time with this.

☐ Someone who will let me think out loud.

☐ Someone who will not tell other people about what I say or do.

☐ Someone who will not think I am crazy because of what I am thinking.

☐ Someone who will be okay with me repeating myself.

☐ Someone who won't tell me what I should do.

☐ Someone who will do some things with me, so I can get a break from this.

☐ Someone who will see me as a good person, no matter what.

☐ Someone who will let me know if I am bothering them.

☐ Someone who will be honest with me.

☐ Someone who will take on some tasks I have trouble doing right now.

☐ Someone who won't let me become inactive.

☐ Someone who will hold me.

☐ Someone who won't get more emotional than me about these things.

☐ Someone who has time for me.

☐ Someone who knew me before all this happened.

☐ Someone who can see that I want to change for the better.

☐ Someone who will help me learn.

List any other characteristics that would be helpful in an expert companion:

☐ Someone who _____.

☐ Someone who _____.

Doing this exercise hopefully clarified the kind of person who could be an expert companion for you. It also may have given you some ideas for how to express your needs to an expert companion. People often need help in figuring out how to help.

You may be thinking, *Wow! Where do I find a person like this?* Alternatively, you may be thinking of just such a person who is already a companion to you. Or perhaps you are at neither extreme but are somewhere in the middle, thinking that you could have someone like this in your life but are not really sure who it would be. So now that you have a better picture of who you would like to have in your life, you can consider who this person or these people could be.

EXERCISE: Finding an Expert Companion

Think of some people from the past who have had some of the characteristics you checked off in the previous exercise. These people might have helped you, or they may have helped others, and you saw how they were able to provide expert companionship. See if you can come up with a few possibilities.

Name: _____

How they helped me or helped others: _____

_____

Name: _____

How they helped me or helped others: _____

_____

Name: _____

How they helped me or helped others: _____

_____

Name: _____

How they helped me or helped others: _____

_____

Now switch to the present time. Think of some people who have reached out to you with compassion or have done something unexpected and helpful. These could be friends or family members, or they may be people whom you do not know well. They may have surprised you with their care, but you have not considered accepting their help, because you do not currently have a strong relationship with them. Write down the names of these people and how they have helped. If you have difficulty identifying anyone, we will come back to this topic later in this chapter.

Name: _____

How they helped me or helped others: _____

_____

Name: _____

How they helped me or helped others: _____

_____

Name: _____

How they helped me or helped others: _____

_____

Name: _____

How they helped me or helped others: _____

_____

By now you may have a better idea of someone you can invite into your current life as an expert companion.

_____

Some people are quite comfortable with asking people to help them, and others are not. Here is an exercise that will help you assess how easy or hard this is for you.

EXERCISE: Inviting People to Be Expert Companions

Place a check mark next to each statement that matches what you believe to be true about yourself.

- ☐ *I can ask for help pretty easily. (+)*
- ☐ *I like to feel independent. (-)*
- ☐ *I think that other people feel good when they get to help others. (+)*
- ☐ *I like to do things my own way. (-)*
- ☐ *I get embarrassed when I am emotional. (-)*
- ☐ *I don't like other people to know I am having trouble. (-)*
- ☐ *I am usually part of a close network of people. (+)*
- ☐ *I enjoy helping others. (-)*
- ☐ *I feel much more comfortable helping than being helped. (-)*
- ☐ *People I know would be hurt if they found out that I didn't let them know I was in need. (+)*
- ☐ *I am hesitant to tell other people what I am feeling or thinking. (-)*
- ☐ *People I know are very warm and compassionate. (+)*
- ☐ *I have seen the people I know offer help to others. (+)*
- ☐ *It is important to me that I look strong and capable. (-)*
- ☐ *I think people would lose respect for me if they saw my vulnerability. (-)*
- ☐ *I have a solid network of friends. (+)*
- ☐ *I am not afraid to show my feelings. (+)*

☐   *I don't trust that people will really follow through with help or stick with me.* (-)

☐   *People often make promises, but few really keep them.* (-)

☐   *I don't embarrass easily.* (+)

☐   *I feel that I am well liked.* (+)

☐   *I have felt betrayed in the past by people I trusted.* (-)

☐   *People have come through for me in surprising ways.* (+)

Scoring: Add up the statements that you checked with a positive sign at the end, and add up the statements that you checked with a negative sign at the end. If the positives are more frequent than the negatives, you will probably be able to seek some of the companionship you need easily. If, on the other hand, you checked the negative items more frequently than you checked the positive items, it may be harder for you to approach someone for help or to accept help when offered. If the positives and negatives are fairly even, you may be conflicted about seeking companionship.

This exercise gives only a general sense of what might make it easy or hard for you to accept companionship. However, it can show you how you may need to start thinking differently in order to benefit from expert companionship.

You may have discovered that you will need more than one person for companionship. This is because some helpers are better at certain things than others. Also, it can be helpful to have more than one expert companion, so you do not call on any one person too often when you are in need. Spreading around your needs for assistance may be more comfortable for you and for them.

How to Ask for Help

This book has emphasized that facing up to the difficult aspects of your situation will make you stronger. If you tend to avoid asking for help or personal closeness in your relationships, this may be your opportunity for you to grow in this area of your life. Connection with others will not only help you deal with trauma but also produce a richer life going forward. So we want you to commit to a plan for finding an expert companion. The next exercise is designed to help you with this.

EXERCISE: A Plan for Help

Identify those people around you whom you can ask for help but you hesitate to approach or don't want to ask. Describe your reasons for not asking until now. Then make a plan to overcome your reluctance, stating the specific actions you will take and when you will take them. Then describe how things went, paying particular attention to those things that surprised you. Look at the example and then write out your own plan in the space that follows. If you have more than one person in mind, make a plan to approach this additional person (or people) as well. You can do this for as many people as you have in mind.

Example:

1. Who is someone you can ask for help? *My friend Julia.*

2. Why haven't you asked this person for help? *Julia has a lot of her own problems. I haven't wanted to burden her and make her life more difficult. Plus, I wasn't sure she would really understand why I'm struggling the way I am.*

3. What is your plan for how you will ask this person for help? Describe the specific actions you will take and when you will take them. Be sure to identify what you need help with.

Date: *October 1.* Action: *Before talking with her, I will write out exactly what I need from her.*

Date: *October 7.* Action: *I will ask her to go to lunch.*

Date: *No later than October 20.* Action: *We will have lunch together and I will ask her for what I need.*

Date: *The day after our lunch.* Action: *I will call her and thank her for talking/listening to me.*

Outcome: *She told me she was honored that I asked her for help. This surprised me. She also said her sister experienced something similar years ago. She always felt guilty that she couldn't help her sister more. I think she may see helping me as a way to make up for what she wasn't able to do for her sister.*

Your plan:

1. Who is someone you can ask for help?

    _____

2. Why haven't you asked this person for help?

    _____

    _____

    _____

    _____

3. What is your plan for how you will ask this person for help? Describe the specific actions you will take and when you will take them. Be sure to identify what you need help with.

    Date: _____ Action: _____

    _____

    Date: _____ Action: _____

    _____

    Date: _____ Action: _____

    _____

    Date: _____ Action: _____

    _____

    Date: _____ Action: _____

    _____

Outcome:

_____

_____

_____

In completing this exercise, we hope that you have begun to see that there are possibilities for some companionship among a variety of people you know. If you've been reluctant to ask for assistance, you may have found that it has do with pride, maintaining your reputation, fear of rejection, or any number of motives. These kinds of motives are very human but may be based on inaccurate thinking. Perhaps you have started to notice flaws in these thoughts and how taking action tests these ideas. Although not everyone you approach for expert companionship will be able to offer just what you want, we hope you will be able to see that some aspects of assistance are worth taking the risk of asking for.

Other Sources of Expert Companionship

If you had trouble in the earlier exercises identifying who could be an expert companion in your life, there are other ways to find this kind of companionship. This section focuses on alternative places to look.

Online Companions

Many people decide to go online to seek expert companions who may be better able to understand their situation than the people around them. You can connect online with others who have been or are going through similar circumstances. You may feel like you don't have to explain yourself so much, because they already know what your feelings and thoughts about the traumatic situation might be. Finding other trauma survivors can give you hope as well as ideas for how to cope. You may find blogs or websites devoted to your particular trauma, and engage in chats. One of the advantages of this form of support for many people is that they can be quite anonymous. This can seem important if you are dealing with a traumatic circumstance that carries some stigma. Finding others online who are in a similar situation solves this problem in two ways. First, they will be less likely to be judgmental. Second, because the communication is anonymous, you will be less anxious about how others might view you.

Inspirational Sources of Expert Companionship

You may struggle with the feeling that no one understands what you've been through. Autobiographical accounts of trauma, through blogs, books, or other media, can be very helpful in reducing the sense of aloneness and the feeling of being an outsider that can come with experiencing trauma. When you suddenly feel removed from the social group to which you have always belonged, because you have experienced something that others do not understand, it is often good to hear from people who have already been traveling the path that you are on. Another source of comfort may be in scripture and your religious faith, where you have a sense that God is your expert companion.

It is important to add that there will always be some aspect of your experience that is unique. However close another's experience may be to yours and however understanding an expert companion may be, there is an essential loneliness in these circumstances that cannot be entirely escaped. You need to understand this so that you will not be unnecessarily disappointed in the efforts expert companions may make. They cannot take the pain from you, and they cannot understand everything.

Professional Companions

Another option for expert companionship is finding a professional companion or helper. There may be a nonprofit organization in your community that provides support to trauma survivors who are specifically in your situation. Some organizations provide individual or group counseling services, and the people who provide the services have a great deal of knowledge about what to expect when dealing with the circumstances that you face. In this way, they may be particularly helpful, because they are used to helping many others whose circumstances are similar to yours.

It may be harder to find an individual psychologist or counselor who is right for you unless you can find someone with a good deal of experience dealing with your particular trauma. You can ask for recommendations from people you know. If you do not know anyone who has worked with a mental health professional, you can contact your local or state professional association for psychologists and counselors, which may be able to give a referral. You can also find referrals through the websites of the American Psychological Association, the American Counseling Association, or *Psychology Today* magazine.

The quality of the relationship a professional offers may be more important than the particular experience that person has with your trauma. If you go to a mental health professional, be clear that you are looking for emotional support in the form of an expert companion. Bear in mind that many mental health professionals are used to working with people who are diagnosed with particular mental disorders whereas you are dealing with trauma. You may be experiencing strong emotions, but this does not mean that you have a mental disorder. If you are sad, you may not be depressed. So it is useful to talk with a professional who understands what you need and can serve as an expert companion, keeping the focus on the kind of relationship that would be most helpful to you. You will know if a professional helper is right for you through your own emotional reaction to being with him or her. You can trust yourself to know.

You Can Be an Expert Companion

You may find yourself becoming an expert companion. It can happen online or in person. It may happen when you meet someone who has been going through a similar circumstance. You may find that you can help each other. This happens as you compare your experiences and perhaps provide each other with new ideas for how to cope. There may be a sense of relief from not having to explain everything to the other person, because your experiences are so similar. But you might find yourself offering expert companionship to people who are facing circumstances very different from yours as well. Being helped by an expert companion may fill you with a sense of gratitude and inspire you to offer this to someone else.

Your ability to be an expert companion will likely evolve as you travel the path toward healing and growth in the aftermath of your trauma. You may not set out to be helpful, and you may find it hard to imagine that in your difficulty you can offer much to anyone else. But as we have suggested, being an expert companion is most essentially a human skill; it is simply providing a presence in these difficult times. Almost anyone can do this. It does not require a professional degree.

Becoming an expert companion is also a route to posttraumatic growth. Here's how it works. Your own experience with trauma becomes a basis for helping others. You perhaps will feel a special affinity for others who have gone through similar circumstances and feel especially compassionate and empathic toward them. Helping others through similar circumstances could even become a mission for you. This could be very rewarding and open up new possibilities in your life that you would never have considered before.

There are possible pitfalls, however, that are worth considering. One is retraumatization. If you are trying to be helpful to someone who is having difficulty, what they tell you about their troubles may add to the struggle you are already having with your own circumstances. This may be a sign that you are not quite ready to be an expert companion and, for the time being, it may be better to focus more on managing your own emotional difficulties. It is also important not to assume that you are similar to another person simply because your circumstances are similar. It can be easy to overidentify, taking over another person's trauma experience and making it your own. Unfortunately, this can lead to assuming you know what is right for someone else.

Another pitfall to expert companionship with other trauma survivors is that it may keep you from being with other people who have not had such experiences. It can become easy to divide the world into the people who have known traumas like yours and people who have not, especially when connecting with others in similar circumstances can be so satisfying and when you find you have expert companionship to offer. You may find at first that your most comfortable relationships are with people who can most easily share your pain. But ultimately you will need to be able to find ways to be close to people who do not have direct experience with circumstances like yours.

Despite these pitfalls, most people find that providing expert companionship to others who are struggling is very rewarding. It can be an unexpected benefit to surviving your trauma.

Things to Remember About Expert Companionship

In this chapter, you have learned about the importance of expert companionship and how expert companionship may meet your needs at this point in time. You've also learned about how to find expert companions, and you've come up with a plan to seek out an expert companion or companions for yourself. We've also encouraged you to consider becoming a particularly effective expert companion yourself—if not now, then in the future after you have taken more steps on the path toward growth.

Here are a few more things to keep in mind. What you need from an expert companion may change over time, and you may find yourself gravitating toward different people in order to meet different needs. For example, you may have someone who is especially comforting to you when you just need a companion to cry with, while another person is more adept at engaging you in conversation about your experiences or about changes in your beliefs. Another companion may be someone who you just like to spend time with, doing things together that can provide a bit of distraction and relief from the hard emotional work of posttraumatic growth.

It is also useful to remember that your expert companions may need a break from being with you at times, so be charitable toward them. You will also need to be able to count on yourself as a good companion. People cannot always be there to help you in times of need, and you will have to rely on your own ability to manage your emotions. You can use the methods we have described in this book (see chapter 3). Finally, be compassionate toward yourself, and keep in mind that posttraumatic growth is hard work, and it takes time.

CHAPTER 7

Finding Meaning, Purpose, and Mission

This chapter challenges you to develop a clearer and perhaps new sense of purpose that extends beyond yourself and your own needs. Engaging in a mission to help others can produce posttraumatic growth in any of the areas we've talked about. By being of service to others, you will become familiar again with your own personal strength and what you have to offer. The satisfaction you feel may give you a greater appreciation of life and perhaps your own life situation, even with its difficulties. You will be exploring new possibilities for yourself, perhaps even new commitments, work, devotions, or personal identity. By engaging in a mission that benefits others, you very likely will feel more compassion and empathy, which will improve your relationships with others. Finally, there is a spiritual aspect to such work that may challenge your beliefs in this area of your life.

This may be a difficult chapter, as it requires considerable self-reflection, challenging of self-defeating behaviors, and taking risks. But almost everyone is able to make this important transition in a journey toward growth. You have to trust in your abilities and sense of compassion. If you have lost your sense of purpose in life, you can get it back or, more likely, develop a changed sense of purpose. Trauma is full of loss, and this may be the most profound loss of all. But taking on this particular challenge of trauma can yield some of the most satisfying aspects of posttraumatic growth.

Loss of Purpose

A particularly cruel aspect of trauma is that it seems to close down parts of your life that have been important and meaningful. This leads to a profound sense of loss and purpose. For example, Mary, a mother who tragically lost her five-year-old son in a car accident, became paralyzed with feelings of loss and grief. Even though she had completed college and begun her career as a nurse, she had always known that her focus in life would be as a mother. When her child was born, Mary left her career and put everything into being a mother. She loved being a mother and thrived in this role. After her son's death, many months went by, and Mary struggled with intense feelings of loss. She told friends and family how empty she felt and how life no longer had meaning. She fell into a deep depression, and her marriage was on the verge of being over. Fortunately, at the request of her friend and former coworker, Mary agreed to visit a support group provided by her local hospice organization. In this group, Mary was able to process her feelings of loss. Over time, her depression lessened and her marriage improved. She and her husband had two more children together, and Mary once again thrived. She also organized support groups for parents who were struggling with the death of a child. Since she found the support group helpful to her in the past, she wanted to help other parents deal with their grief and learn to really live again.

Mary is a good example of how loss and grief can cause someone to lose a sense of meaning and purpose. In fact, for Mary, her new purpose in life seemed to be one of grieving. It was difficult for her to see beyond the despair she was in. She was unable to see new possibilities or other pathways. This is a point in the growth process where some people get stuck. In essence, loss and grief can blind you to new possibilities and pathways. These feelings can simply take over. Fortunately for Mary, she found a way past these obstacles and ultimately found new meaning in her role as a parent and in the work she does in serving other bereaved parents.

Managing Loss and Grief

In chapter 3, we talked about how to manage strong emotions and intrusive ruminations. The concepts we discussed and exercises we shared are relevant here. However, if you continue to struggle with loss and grief, there are some other things you can do to manage these feelings.

It's important to understand that strong feelings of loss and grief are normal after enduring a difficult life event. These feelings are common not only after a death, as with Mary, but also in the aftermath of many traumatic life events, as trauma always involves loss in some way. Whether you lost a loved one to illness or an accident, had your sense of safety and security stolen from you after being assaulted, or were left feeling vulnerable, worthless, and unloved after a breakup or divorce, it will take time to heal. Feeling depressed and anxious, having problems with sleep and appetite, and feeling angry, resentful, and numb are to be expected. It doesn't mean you are crazy. And for the vast majority of people, these problems are time-limited.

Remind yourself that healing takes time. Although time does not necessarily heal all wounds, in spite of what the old saying claims, it certainly does help. What is important in this period of time is what you do with it. Don't rush through the grieving process. Allow time to take away the acute distress associated with loss while also understanding that some degree of longing and loss may remain. Accept the fact that your life has changed while also remembering that growth can come with change.

Don't forget to rely on those around you who care about you and whom you trust. Few things in life are done well in isolation. This is particularly true for overcoming emotional struggle. The collective compassion and wisdom of those around you is immense. Tap into it by asking for help. In addition to asking for emotional support, you can ask for help with grocery shopping, cooking, cleaning, and having someone go on walks with you. It is critical that you take care of your basic needs like nutrition, physical activity, and maintaining your home.

Lastly, let yourself mourn. Grief can produce a profound sense of emptiness and despair. In order to overcome these feelings, you need to actively mourn your loss. You can actively mourn the death of a loved one through a wake, a funeral, or a memorial service. These formal activities allow you to remember your loved one and start the process of living without your loved one physically present. Of course, such rituals are only a start, and many more actions over time can help you mourn. But how do you mourn other losses? It depends on who you are and what you have lost.

For someone who has recently divorced, an act of mourning could be donating to charity anything that an ex-spouse chose to leave behind. Or it could consist of burying, burning, or giving away pictures and other visual reminders of the relationship. A person who narrowly escaped death from a motor vehicle accident may hold a "funeral" mourning the loss of her previous sense of safety and security while also celebrating the promise for creating a more realistic yet optimistic view of life. Again, it depends on the person and the trauma. An activity we've found helpful when working with people who are struggling in the aftermath of trauma is to ask them to become the professional. The ability to look outward and to focus on providing support, guidance, and advice to others is a great way to temporarily separate yourself from your distress. It also promotes insight into ways you can move past your own stuck points.

EXERCISE: Being the Therapist

Assume you are a psychologist, counselor, or social worker who has been asked to help Erin, whose story follows. Read the story and then answer the questions in the space provided.

> Late one evening, after walking back to her car in a shopping mall parking lot, Erin was pulled into a van against her will. She was beaten, raped, and tossed out on the side of the road and left to die. Erin now leaves her apartment only to attend classes and to go grocery shopping. She avoids spending time with her friends and rarely calls her parents anymore. She ruminates about the assault and believes she can never trust another man. At some level, she believes that the life she has known is over and she is destined to live a sad and fearful life.

1. What would you say or do to help Erin understand the emotions she is currently experiencing?

   _____

   _____

   _____

2. How would you help Erin understand the process of grief? What are some ways she can start to overcome her intense feelings of loss?

   _____

   _____

   _____

3. What advice can you give Erin that will help her reach out to others? How can she make a plan to do this?

_____

_____

_____

4. What are some of the potential losses she may feel as a result of her assault? And what are some ways in which she can mourn those losses?

_____

_____

_____

5. Assuming Erin has made progress in dealing with her feelings of loss and grief, what do you believe would be the next steps in her journey toward growth?

_____

_____

_____

6. Does thinking about Erin's situation provide insight into what to do about your own sense of loss and grief?

_____

_____

_____

7. Do you believe the guidance and advice you provided Erin would work for you? If so, in what ways? If not, why not?

_____

_____

_____

8. Who in your life can help you deal with your loss and grief and help you explore new possibilities in life? Who are they and how would they be helpful? (You might return to chapter 6 to identify possible expert companions.)

_____

_____

_____

We hope that this exercise helped you recognize some ways to manage your own feelings of loss and grief. Sometimes it helps to take a step back from your own situation.

_____

Taking a step back from your own struggles and focusing on the struggles of others may help you gain clarity. It also reinforces the important process of serving others in their time of need, as others have been of help to us.

A Path to New Possibilities

Life meaning and purpose is not something that is stumbled upon or that you just wake up to one morning and magically possess. It can be difficult to imagine what new possibilities and pathways are available or what would make life richer. But meaning and purpose are not so much discovered as created. Instead of waiting for them to come to you, you have to seek them out. It takes creativity.

To start, it will help to focus on the value of what you have rather than on what the trauma has taken from you. We acknowledge that this may seem Pollyannaish, naive, or overly optimistic. However, the reality is that trauma is something that happened to you. The trauma is not who you are or what defines you. You are a complex individual, and there is a lot more to who you are as a person. We concede that it may be difficult to value those things that gave you satisfaction and meaning in your life before you experienced trauma. After trauma, you may still have many of those things in your life, but your perspective has shifted. As noted earlier in the book, trauma is akin to an earthquake that shakes the foundation of how you see yourself. That's why many trauma survivors find it helpful to ask for the perspectives of others.

Who better to help you identify your blind spots than someone who knows you, cares about you, and can be honest with you? And what is more powerful, therapeutic, or freeing than knowing that someone close to you recognizes your value, worth, and goodness in spite of what happened to you? Other people can help you remember what motivated you and kept you going before the trauma. The trick is to identify those people who are most likely to be of help and then seek out their assistance. It may be someone you have already identified as an expert companion, or it may be someone you haven't yet considered. It may be several people, or it may be only one. It may be someone who may not know you well but is someone you know to be honest, insightful, and caring.

This next exercise will take someone else's perspective to help you see what you have in your life that you can still be grateful for.

EXERCISE: Finding Gratitude

Think of someone who would be able to identify those things in your life that provided you with meaning, purpose, worth, and satisfaction before your trauma. Then answer the questions.

1. Who is this person in your life?

---

2. What are five things this person would likely say you should be grateful for?

_____

_____

_____

_____

_____

3. For each of those five things, what would the person say that would possibly interfere with your being thankful? What are some obstacles in the way?

    1. _____

    2. _____

    3. _____

    4. _____

    5. _____

We hope this exercise helped you to see that there are things in your life to be grateful for. Sometimes it just takes looking at things from a different perspective.

Gratitude is defined simply as being thankful. It is the ability to appreciate what you or others have and the ability to give and receive kindness. Sometimes stepping outside of yourself can help you see what you can still be grateful for.

Next we'd like you to engage in some self-reflection to identify some possible areas for finding greater meaning and purpose.

The Path Behind

Hindsight may or may not actually be 20/20, but it can be revealing. Again, feelings of loss and grief make it difficult to fully appreciate those things in your life that have given you meaning and purpose. You've basically lost focus. One way to regain that focus is to reconsider your past. If you deliberately spend time reflecting on what your life was like before the trauma, then you are likely to identify various people, places, and things that gave you meaning. Maybe it was the desire to further your education or learn a trade. Maybe it was a relationship that was growing or on the mend but which got sidetracked because of the trauma. The next exercise will assist you in remembering.

EXERCISE: Looking Back

Think back to your life prior to your trauma and then answer the questions in the space provided:

1. Who in your life provided meaning and purpose?

    _____

2. Are these people still a source of meaning and purpose in your life? If not, can anything be done to change this?

    _____

    _____

3. What things (experiences, places, possessions, and so on) in your life provided meaning and purpose?

    _____

4. Are they still a source of meaning and purpose in your life? If not, can anything be done to change this?

_____

_____

A deliberate, compassionate, and thoughtful self-reflection about the past can help you uncover what has been hidden.

_____

The Path Ahead

Instead of looking into the past, now we want you to peer into your crystal ball. Spend some time imagining what your life would look like if you could write your life story. What people, places, or things would you like to write into your life that would give you meaning and purpose? Be creative and don't limit yourself. You are the story-teller and have complete control over the narrative. If you find this activity difficult, don't worry. Creating a new life narrative will be covered in more detail in the final chapter. This exercise will help you get started.

_____

EXERCISE: Looking Forward

Envision what your life will look like in the future and answer the questions in the space provided.

1. What people would you like to have in your future who can provide meaning and purpose for you?

_____

_____

2. Why would these people be a source of meaning and purpose for you?

_____

_____

3. What can you do to bring these people into your life?

_____

_____

4. What things (experiences, places, possessions, and so on) would you like to have in your future that can provide meaning and purpose for you?

_____

_____

5. Why would they be a source of meaning and purpose for you?

_____

_____

6. What can you do to bring these things into your life?

_____

_____

Now is the time to consider what your future will look like and what you will need. Being able to identify this puts you in a great position to live a full and rewarding life. Even if you don't have a sense of meaning and purpose now, imagining what your future can look like is a step toward getting there.

The Path Never Taken

Each and every one of us can look back on our life and identify missed opportunities. Sometimes we may tell ourselves we'll come back to it later, and other times we make a choice while not fully understanding its impact. Regardless of the reasons, the past is full of possibilities that were never seized. This next exercise will help you explore if you could benefit from rediscovering those paths never taken.

EXERCISE: A Different Direction

Take an honest appraisal of those things in your past that, if acted on now or in the future, would potentially provide you with meaning and purpose. Then answer the questions in the space provided.

1. Were there opportunities in your life to connect with someone who would have enriched your life, but for some reason you chose not to establish a connection? If so, who was that person? Why did you decide not to connect with this person?

    _____

    _____

    _____

    _____

2. Could you connect with this person now or in the future? If so, how would you go about it?

    _____

    _____

    _____

    _____

3. Were there any missed opportunities to participate in activities, relationships, or endeavors that you could consider now or in the future? If so, what were they, and why did you decide not to pursue these things?

_____

_____

_____

_____

4. Are the opportunities to pursue these things available to you now or possibly available in the future?

_____

_____

_____

_____

This exercise asked you to look back at paths never taken and explore why you didn't go in certain directions. Sometimes revisiting missed opportunities can bring new meaning and purpose to your life.

Finding new possibilities for growth takes careful consideration. It also requires you to be patient with yourself and to show self-compassion. We understand how easy it is to be critical of things you've done or not done. We also know that reflecting on the past can be associated with painful memories. We ask that you do your best to push aside those hurtful memories and focus instead on what life has given you and can give you now. What are you thankful for? What people in your life build you up? Are there unfinished parts of the past that would enrich your life now? These are all questions you must ask yourself and those around you who know and care about you.

Identifying the Mission

Once you are able to identify areas of potential growth, you can focus your efforts on developing a sense of mission. Some refer to having a mission as altruism, or acting for others. It's the process of putting the needs of others ahead of your own, which in turn provides meaning and purpose for yourself. You can also look at it as the process of developing service-oriented goals.

Finding meaning and purpose in your life doesn't necessarily have to be altruistic or service oriented. For example, a strong spiritual or religious connection could provide meaning and purpose in your life. However, as part of that spiritual or religious connection, you could also decide that your purpose and meaning comes not just from this connection but also from a desire to help others find spiritual or religious meaning too. In our experience, most people find that placing service to others at the core of their personal growth gives them the greatest satisfaction.

As you navigate the process of posttraumatic growth, we want you to consider a few questions. Does serving others fit within your life goals? Does it seem to align with how you see yourself or how you believe others see you? What are the benefits and limitations of putting the needs of others along with or in front of your own? Once you can answer these questions, you will be well beyond where most people exist.

We will lead you through some steps that can help you to develop a service-oriented way of interacting with people, or a mission that will benefit others. Even a small step in this direction will enable you to experience posttraumatic growth. Here are some questions to help you reflect on who in your life could be a model of service and mission, someone who has been down this path already.

EXERCISE: Finding Models of Service and Mission

Name some people who have been models of service and mission for you in these different parts of your life.

From your childhood and adolescence: _____

_____

Family members: _____

_____

Teachers: _____

_____

Religious figures: _____

_____

Neighbors: _____

_____

Coaches: _____

_____

Friends: _____

_____

Families of friends: _____

_____

Business people: _____

_____

Police officers or others in authority: _____

_____

Name any others that don't fit into the above list: _____

_____

Name some people present in your life now who are models of service to others:

_____

_____

_____

Now choose someone from the list you just made and describe as specifically as possible what that person did that you consider a service or a mission. Consider the actions—behaviors, activities, or commitments—that defined that service.

Person: _____

_____

_____

_____

_____

Mission or service: _____

_____

_____

_____

_____

Specific actions: _____

_____

_____

_____

_____

The purpose of this exercise was to get you thinking about what you could do to create a new sense of purpose. Having a mission like the people you described may seem foreign to you. If so, you might think of talking with them, if possible, about their motives in engaging in good works and how they discovered ways to do this.

_____

Be aware that there are many people who have missions that you would not know about. It's possible to give anonymously. Consider the following story.

Emily is a businesswoman who travels the same route each day to work. This route takes her past a small park that gets little use. On many days, she noticed a man in the park who was often sitting at a picnic table reading a book. He was poorly dressed and always alone. One day, she noticed he was not at the table, and she decided to walk into the park to see if he was okay. She soon spotted the same man sitting outside a shabby tent near the back of the park. He was clearly homeless. She kept at a distance and did not think he saw her. She decided she would like to help him but was wary about approaching. She left the park and thought about what to do. She decided that each day as she drove by, she would check to see if the man was at the table and would leave something for him if he were not there. On her way to work, she would carry something with her and just leave it at the table when he wasn't there. On various occasions, she left clothing, food, and books. She thought of herself as his secret benefactor. She enjoyed the idea that all he knew was that some kind person was out there who noticed him and showed some caring and compassion.

The next exercise will help you identify your own mission. You may be able to help people you know well or people with whom you have only passing contact. Or like Mary, whom you met at the beginning of this chapter, you may wish to help others who have gone through experiences similar to yours.

EXERCISE: Identifying Your Mission

Identify people whom you have some contact with in daily life and whom you might be able to assist in some way. You can include other living beings besides people or other things of importance to you that could be involved in a service or mission that you define. Name these people or things in the different parts of your life listed here.

At work: _____

_____

At school: _____

_____

In the neighborhood: _____

_____

Family: _____

_____

Friends: _____

_____

On the Internet: _____

_____

At stores and businesses: _____

_____

Other people or things of possible importance in your daily environment: _____

_____

Are there certain people whom you identify with or empathize with because of your trauma?

_____

_____

Now choose someone or something from the list you just made and describe as specifically as possible what you might be able to do that you consider a service or a mission. Name the actions—specific behaviors, activities, or commitments—that would define your service.

Person or focus of service: _____

_____

_____

_____

Mission or service: _____

_____

_____

_____

Specific actions to take: _____

_____

_____

_____

These ideas could be small steps to take to start a process of living with a greater sense of purpose, or they could be great challenges for you. Sometimes it is good to have a mixture of both, so that you define for yourself short-term and long-term goals.

A Commitment to Serve

A newfound sense of purpose is unlikely to suddenly appear as you begin to pursue your mission but is more likely to develop over time. It will be important to commit to an activity or set of activities for at least several weeks before you evaluate how this may be affecting you. That said, it's also important to be flexible about this process. Think of this as exploring possibilities. Your commitment should be to explore and create your purpose and to test out missions of service. Your missions can evolve over time as new possibilities present themselves. You are likely to find your possibilities increasing as you engage people in your attempts to serve. And as you do so, you will most likely discover that you got more out of it than you believe you have given.

CHAPTER 8

Your New Life Story

The stress of trauma has presented you with some challenges in living but also forced you to consider what your life will be like going forward. In this workbook, you have learned strategies to manage the emotional distress that comes with this disruption in your life. You have also learned that one of the most difficult challenges is that you must consider or reconsider what you believe about the most fundamental aspects of living life well: what kind of person you are, what kind of world you live in, what makes sense and is meaningful to you, and what your future will be. In chapter 7, you focused on finding ways to live a life of importance. You developed some principles that will sustain you into the future and some missions that will benefit others as well as yourself.

In this chapter, you will integrate all of this change into a coherent story of your life. What you have been going through may have been quite profound and represents a new pathway and new principles. It is important to see how this came about and how it relates to your previous ways of living, the traumatic stress you have encountered, and the struggle with this stress that you have engaged in. If you think that such changes and your future happen by magic, are simply random, or are even destined to be, it will be harder to sustain these positive changes. But if you understand the logic of what has been happening in your life, these changes will be integrated into a life story that makes more sense and will be easier to sustain. You will have the sense of knowing that you are making things happen rather than having things just happening to you.

Seeing New Possibilities

Making plans is something most people like to do. Children often have a sense of what they will be when they grow up, although their plans usually change over time. Most adults also make plans about what they wish to accomplish, and sometimes this works well. However, events can insert surprising twists into the story that you think you are living. You can think that you are constructing a life story that makes sense and is important, but somewhere you find that it lacks meaning. As a result, your life story may change in surprising ways. This change often occurs after a period of struggle, uncertainty, and sometimes experimentation. Traumatic events are particularly powerful in knocking you off the trajectory you have set for yourself.

With such change come opportunities for reconsidering how to live: new priorities, principles, and goals. Being able to see new possibilities is an aspect of posttraumatic growth. How do new possibilities arise? Sometimes they arise because of things that make the old way of living impossible. Sometimes survivors of trauma have to do something novel just to manage their situation. Sometimes a change in core beliefs forces a change in behavior. Again and again, in the lives of people we've known, we have seen how the story can change. Here is how a thirty-one-year-old man named Barry described his life story and how it altered.

Barry's Life Story

"I was working in a paper bag factory. I was a young guy, enjoying life, drinking a lot, and pretty much carefree. There was this old guy, about fifty-five or sixty, I guess, doing the same crummy job I was, and I came in real hungover one day. He hadn't ever said much to me. I'd been working there almost a year, and he more or less grunted at me. Wasn't the friendly type. Seemed like a loner or something. So anyway, I came in hungover one day—and it wasn't the first time.

"So I was eating something out of my lunch box, and next thing I know, he's standing over me. He says, 'Barry, right?' I tell him, 'Yeah, I'm Barry.' I was surprised he knew my name. He says, 'I've been watching you.' I didn't know what he meant, but it didn't sound good. So he says, 'I've been watching you, and you're in trouble.' I'm figuring maybe I screwed up something on the job, and I can't figure out what, but he goes on. He says, 'You're screwing up your life, son. What are you doing here? You go out drinking at night with your buddies, come back here in the morning all hungover, day after day, and getting nowhere. You'd better get it together before you find yourself as old as me and have nothin'. Better look at yourself and where you are. That's where you're headed.' Then he turned and walked away.

"First I thought, *Screw him, what does he know?* And I went back to eating my crummy sandwich. Then I looked at that sandwich, some bologna and white bread and mustard, and I looked around at the factory, dirty and loud, and I thought about how I felt coming to work and what I was going to do after. And I looked at him walking away, kind of hunched over and alone. I wondered what his story was, and started to think, *What if that is me in another twenty or thirty years? I don't want that to be my story, but right now, maybe it is.*

"So I finished my shift and went out with the guys later like usual. Had my usual beer. Talked about the usual stuff. But I was kind of detached, sort of observing myself doing all this, and it was like I was in a movie and I was acting out this movie or something. And when I was looking at it that way, it was a pretty pathetic story. It all seemed pointless. Kind of embarrassing. I started thinking about what my parents raised me for—*Was it this?* I couldn't enjoy myself. I went home early. I felt depressed and tried to put the day out of my mind. I was pissed off with that guy at work—he was messing me up. But I couldn't ignore what he'd said. I had trouble sleeping."

What is perhaps most striking about what Barry said is that he thought of this encounter in terms of stories: the man's, his own, and the fact that stories can change. It is also striking that this man, virtually a stranger, took ten seconds to say something that had an impact. It started Barry thinking, rethinking his own life story that he was writing. He became aware that he was writing this life story by living it the way he was. He also became aware that it was not a good story, and he did not want it to continue in the way the old man's story had. Somehow, the man had taken him by surprise, and this kind of surprise is what people sometimes need to make them take notice of things they have previously missed. When you start noticing things, and when you start to question the story you are living out, and when you notice what has happened in another life story, all kinds of new possibilities can arise.

Another striking thing about Barry's story is that once these questions were triggered, he couldn't stop thinking about them. This is an example of intrusive rumination, where you have something on your mind that you can't get away from. This was starting to happen to Barry, and it was pretty unpleasant. But it was also the indication that change was starting. Soon Barry started thinking about his life in a more deliberate way. Doing a life story review is often a useful way to examine your situation, and a very productive way to start thinking about change.

Here is what happened when Barry started to review his life story:

"I started thinking about how I had gotten to this place. I started thinking about the paper bag job. I took it because it was easy for me, and I wanted something easy because I had screwed up things so bad. I had dropped out of college because I didn't want to study. I got an IT job that I screwed up in the same way, and then after my girlfriend dumped me and I had to move out, I had to get a job to make ends meet. My parents wouldn't let me move back in, so here I was in the paper bag place. Pretty pathetic story. And I was making it more pathetic."

Although there is no single event in Barry's story that most people would view as traumatic, there was a series of events that were traumatic in the sense that they challenged his ideas about himself, his future, and what kind of world he was living in—in other words, his core beliefs.

Although questioning your core beliefs can be painful, it is a necessary step in rewriting your life story. You may want to refer back to chapter 2 if you need to review how core beliefs can be affected by trauma. Here is an exercise that will help you understand how Barry began to question his core beliefs.

EXERCISE: Noticing the Examination of Core Beliefs

Play psychologist for a moment as you consider what Barry said about his experiences. Then answer these questions in the space provided.

What event or events in Barry's story represent times when his core beliefs were challenged? At what point did he start to question himself?

1. _____

2. _____

3. _____

4. _____

5. _____

What core beliefs do you think Barry began to question?

_____

_____

_____

_____

_____

If you had difficulty answering these questions, don't worry. The point is just to get you thinking about how core beliefs can be affected by trauma. You may want to come back to this exercise after reading more of Barry's story, which we will return to shortly.

You may have noticed in Barry's story that he had gotten messages from various people that he was on a self-destructive path. The university had told him he was failing, his IT employer had told him he was failing, his girlfriend told him he was failing, and even his parents might have given a similar message by telling him he could not come back to live with them. However, it took a stranger in the factory to get the message across.

You might wonder why. Sometimes it is hard to predict what event will have the biggest impact on someone's life, and certainly it would seem unlikely that a single encounter with a coworker at lunch would provide the main motivation for change. Perhaps it was the pileup of events in Barry's life. Maybe it was the shock of how this man at work had approached him. For some reason, this was the final episode in a series of shocks to his core beliefs that occurred in his tumultuous twenties. He was prompted to rethink these beliefs because they were being contradicted by the life story he was creating. Here is how Barry described it.

"I started thinking back to what I had been doing over the past ten years and how things seemed to have gotten offtrack. I thought I was a smart guy who was going to be successful, meaning make a lot of money. I thought it would come pretty easy because I was smart, attractive, and had a good personality. *Life was going to be fun.* So I did college like it was a done deal and flunked out. But I figured, *No problem, I know enough to get a good job without a degree. In IT, who cares as long as you can do it?* And I was right about that, but I still didn't work, so I got fired from that. Then my girlfriend told me to get out because I was a lazy bum, when I thought that wouldn't happen, because I was such a great guy. Then I figured my parents would help me out—they've got money—but my dad said I was turning into a lazy bum and I had better learn to take care of myself. It was starting to add up—I think I was starting to worry about where all this was going—but I still had my friends to drink with. They liked me—job or no job—and the paper bag place helped me get by. And my buddies thought it was kind of funny, me working there, and it was a joke. So I could get by like that. Then, somehow that guy at the plant showed me it was no joke. This was life. My life. It was turning into his, however he got there. Somehow that unnerved me. I really started to think about all this. I couldn't ignore stuff anymore. It just didn't work."

This story is one example of how people begin to see new possibilities. You can see that a number of events could have been a turning point in Barry's life story, but they didn't have that impact. With each crisis, he was still able to convince himself that things were all right. But the encounter at work started a new process for him. Barry came to a new understanding of his core beliefs and the life story that is based on them. It is important to pay attention to this relationship between what Barry came to believe and the new direction of his life story.

"It is funny how I started to rethink everything once this all got started. First I started thinking I needed a better job. Then I started thinking I needed to drink less. Then I started to think that my friends were putting up with me being a screwup, and I started thinking, *Is that true friendship or not? Maybe good friends don't just accept everything you do.* I had the very weird thought— now this is very weird—that the guy at the factory was a true friend because he called me on it. Now that is weird thinking, right? This guy who seems to want nothing to do with me, just tells me I'm a screwup and walks away, may be a better friend than my drinking buddies?

"And then I started thinking of my ex-girlfriend and my parents, that instead of being angry with them for rejecting me, maybe they were right. Then I started thinking that, no, they were just concerned I wasn't making money—me making money was all they cared about. But maybe not. Then I started thinking, *Maybe I shouldn't care so much about making money.* And actually I hadn't been caring that much. Otherwise, I wouldn't be working in a paper bag factory! So, then, what *should* I care about? Whatever that is, it is going to motivate me going forward. I have to figure out what to care about enough, to do something besides drink and party and just get by. So that's where I am, trying to figure that out and make sure I don't end up with the same story as the old guy in the factory."

Barry's story is a wonderful example of how a challenge to your core beliefs can force you to see new possibilities. The last part—where Barry says he has to figure out what to care about enough, so he can do something different—is very accurate. He's looking for a sense of meaning and purpose.

Can you relate to aspects of Barry's story? Who you are and the events in your life may be very different. But the impact of trauma on your core beliefs, the need to find new meaning and purpose, is something that you probably have experienced too. It is this search for new meaning that shapes your new life story.

Putting It All Together

By now, you are probably ready to put together what you have been working on in this book so far. You can look at the story of your life up to this point, where you have gotten to, and where you seem to be headed into your future. Of course, none of us can guarantee a particular future. Life circumstances can change in ways that are out of our control, and there may very well be more difficulties and traumas ahead that will challenge you. But your task is not only to develop principles, beliefs, and ways of living that will motivate you in a more satisfying future but also to create a path for yourself that can help you to endure future challenges. Some aspects of the story will change, but the basic stuff—your principles and beliefs about what is important—will be sustainable. This can help you meet the challenges ahead.

The first step is to examine your current principles and beliefs about living, the core beliefs we talked about in chapter 2.

EXERCISE: Your Fundamental Principles of Living

First review your responses to the exercise in chapter 2 entitled "A Self-Assessment of the Challenge to Your Core Beliefs." Then in the space provided, write what you have come to believe about these central life issues. If you need more space, you can write in your journal.

1. *The degree to which I believe things that happen to people are fair:*

_____

_____

_____

_____

_____

2. *The degree to which I believe things that happen to people are controllable:*

_____

_____

_____

_____

3. *My beliefs about why other people think and behave the way that they do:*

_____

_____

_____

_____

4. *My beliefs about my relationships with other people:*

_____

_____

_____

_____

_____

5. *My beliefs about my own abilities, strengths, and weaknesses:*

_____

_____

_____

_____

6. *My expectations for my future:*

_____

_____

_____

_____

7.   *My beliefs about the meaning of my life:*

_____

_____

_____

_____

8.   *My spiritual or religious beliefs:*

_____

_____

_____

_____

9.   *My beliefs about my own value or worth as a person:*

_____

_____

_____

_____

YOUR NEW LIFE STORY

Writing about your beliefs may be difficult to do in a few words. You may be still in the process of formulating them. Traumatic life events often confront people with the need to take a hard look at such beliefs for the first time. And since posttraumatic growth is a process, you should not expect to have all this figured out. What is important is that you pay attention to these things. Each of us is a philosopher in a way, trying to figure out how to live well.

_____

Now we want you to consider how these beliefs figure into the way you have lived your life in the past, how you are living now, and how you may live in the future. The next exercise will prompt you to consider the life story you have been living up to now and a possible future that would be consistent with your evolving core beliefs. This exercise will help you start thinking along these lines. Unless you do something differently, where will your story take you?

_____

EXERCISE: Your Developing Life Story

Use the space provided to summarize your story before and after the trauma (writing it out, or drawing it, or using any other format). We understand that the story could go on for many pages, but we're only asking for the overview. If your story involved more than one trauma, focus on the events that triggered you to question your core values. After you've completed these summaries, write out a new post-trauma story. How would you like things to be different? What direction would your life take if you were in control?

Life before the trauma(s): What was the story of your life before the trauma or traumas? What was it like before the interruption of the difficulties you experienced? What did you assume about your life and where you were headed?

_____

_____

_____

_____

_____

_____

_____

_____

_____

_____

_____

_____

_____

_____

_____

_____

_____

_____

_____

_____

You might notice how this story was leading to good things in your life or to bad things. There may be things that were valuable and important, and there may be other things that were leading to some very unfortunate places. What were the core beliefs you were operating on? How did the traumatic events of your life change your direction or perhaps simply stop you in your tracks?

_____

_____

_____

_____

_____

_____

_____

_____

_____

_____

_____

_____

_____

Your current story: Summarize the post-trauma story of your life. What are the core beliefs you are operating on? Describe what your story will look like if nothing were to change and you stayed on the same course you're currently on.

_____

_____

_____

_____

_____

_____

_____

_____

_____

_____

_____

_____

_____

_____

Again, you might notice how this story leads to good things in your life or to bad things. There may be things that you find valuable and important, and there may be things that could lead to some unfortunate places. If this story scares you a little, it's a warning that you need to make some changes. If it's looking like you have some good possibilities in the future, you may already have started on the path toward posttraumatic growth. You might want to include some of these positive things in the story you will be writing next.

Your new story: Summarize the new story of your life. In doing this you can assume for the moment that you are in complete control of how things will turn out. What core beliefs would you wish to express through your life story? How would you like things to be different? How would you incorporate any of these aspects of posttraumatic growth into your story: personal strength, improved relationships, appreciation of life, new possibilities, and spiritual change? Describe below what your story would look like.

_____

_____

_____

_____

_____

_____

_____

_____

_____

_____

_____

_____

_____

_____

_____

_____

_____

_____

_____

_____

_____

_____

_____

_____

_____

The purpose of this exercise is to help you become more aware of how life can be different. Your life can be an expression of new core beliefs and other elements of post-traumatic growth. We want to get you thinking about the possibilities. Maybe you are starting to see that there are a variety of possible post-trauma outcomes that can lead to a more enjoyable and rewarding life. The life story you wrote isn't the only one. The future that you have described for yourself may be only one of the possibilities that might be fulfilling for you. If you can imagine others, you can write about them as well.

We also hope that the difference between your current story and your future story is clear and promising. As the author of your life, are you writing a miserable tale with a horrible ending, or are you constructing a meaningful and purposeful life filled with new possibilities and hope? We believe that the latter is possible. You may have trouble believing in a bright future for yourself right now, but if you keep using the principles you have been practicing while reading this workbook, the possibilities will become clearer.

A Final Story and Some Concluding Thoughts

We want to introduce you to Ryan. He is thirty-two years old with a face permanently scarred from the fire that burned down his house six months ago. With shame and embarrassment, he tells his story.

Ryan's Life Story

"I have always been a drinker. Well, not always. But pretty much since I started, when I was fifteen. See this face? Well, that's where it's got me. Worse than that, though. Before the fire, I never had got in real trouble with drinking. My buddies, we'd go after work and have a few. I liked to have some beer working out in the yard. I got a DUI once, but it didn't get in the way of my work or anything.

"My wife, Tricia, never liked it though, since I would come home after work late being at the bar. She'd say I was getting to be an alcoholic, which seemed ridiculous. I was taking care of business, working and all. But now I can see it was true, that except for being at work, I was pretty much always drinking. Tricia would complain about what the kids were learning from this.

Like, 'Do you want them to grow up to be drunks?' Or she would tell me I always smelled like alcohol. She'd say, 'I'm not interested in having sex with someone whose skin smells like a bar.' She'd worry a lot if she had to go out of town on a business trip. She'd get on my case and say, 'Can I trust you to be sober and take care of the kids?' Beer was getting between us a lot, and I thought she was just being, well, I would say lots of stuff under my breath about her, and I guess I just drank to show her that she was crazy and that I didn't need to stop.

"So, back in May, Tricia was going on a business trip, and we went through this again, and it was a bad one, and I was really fed up with her when she left. I was in a real sour mood. I was nasty to the kids, got them to bed that night early, because I didn't want to deal with them and was feeling real sorry for myself. Thinking *I don't deserve this crap. I'm a grown man and can do what I want. I'm not hurting anybody. No wonder I drink, having to put up with this.* I started thinking about getting divorced. I had thought of that before, but I didn't want to put my kids through that. Never thought of stopping drinking as an option though. So I'm thinking, *I'm trapped. This is my life in this miserable marriage. Just let me have my beer, my friends, enjoy myself a little.* So I'm thinking about all this, and how nice it is my wife is on her trip, and *I've got some peace and can do what I want. So I will take advantage of it and drink what I want. The kids are in bed, and I don't have to worry.*

"I guess I passed out. I don't know, but I'm on the sofa in the living room, and I wake up hearing screaming, and there is smoke all over, and I'm, like, completely out of it, and I can't figure out what is going on. And I get up and stumble and immediately start coughing like crazy from the smoke. I try to get through the kitchen to the kids upstairs, but the kitchen's full of fire. I dive in there trying to get through it, and I get fire on me, and I just run out into the garage.

"I just couldn't do it. I'm so sorry. I tried, but it was too much, and I was still messed up, and I couldn't think straight. And then I heard the sirens. Someone had called. And when they got there, I remember, it was out in the front yard, and I had rolled around to put out the fire, and I was still coughing. They were asking me about anyone else, and I said my kids. Turns out Jack had jumped out the window and was around back with broken legs, but Evie was inside. My God, this was bad. They got in there and got her out unconscious. It's all a blur, my stupid drunk self out there and the firefighters doing their work. They were giving me oxygen and probably had no idea I was still drunk. Neighbors around, concerned for me, trying to comfort me. They got a couple ambulances there and took us all to the hospital.

"So, anyway, the rest of it is that they called Tricia. I couldn't talk to her. I mean, physically I could have, but I was afraid. I knew she would end up furious with me when it all came out. Evie was still not doing well. Tricia got back the next day. I can imagine what hell she went through, trying to get back and worried to death. They kept me in the hospital because of the burns, but I was breathing okay. Jack was going to be okay with his legs, but he was traumatized and so scared. And we talked with the doctors about what is happening with Evie. It's all because of the smoke, no fire was up there, thank God, but she's got some brain damage. Because she's so young, they think she may recover, but they don't know everything about how much. But she's a little fighter, and she's getting better. She's getting a lot of care, rehab therapy, occupational therapy, and those things.

"So, the rest of it is, we got no house right now, but the insurance is getting it rebuilt. I am with my folks and Tricia and the kids are with hers. She can't stand to look at me or talk to me. They did an investigation, and it was some kind of electrical short in the kitchen that started it, but she blames me. She should, because of course, if I wasn't passed out like that, I could have handled the whole thing, and the kids would be okay. I don't care at all about myself and the burns. I feel like I deserve them. I don't know if I'm going to get plastic surgery. We got enough bills, and that's the last thing. I haven't had anything to drink since that night. Beer disgusts me. Makes me think of all this and how I have ruined things."

Six months later, a little over a year after the fire, Ryan is beginning to write a different life story. As you hear this part of Ryan's story, be a good listener, and be thinking of what you have learned about the posttraumatic growth process.

"I'm feeling better. I was suicidal for a while, didn't think I deserved to live after all this. Tricia still thinks of me as a horrible guy who ruined our lives and made my daughter's life into something...well, we don't know what it will be, but it didn't have to be this. So the house is done and up for sale. We're not going back. We're renting a place for her and the kids. I'm still with my folks. Our marriage is over, but at least she is starting to trust me with the kids. Stopping drinking is the big thing. Huge.

"It's strange. They say it is so hard to do and all. But you know, I just have not wanted any. Not at all. I want to leave all that behind. I go to AA meetings every so often, not to make sure I don't drink or anything but just to see some people. And the thing that makes most sense to me is when we talk about living honest and about taking the drinking away so you can see the rest of it, everything else that's messed up. That's what I have been concentrating on—the rest of it. And I think of it, the big thing with me is being selfish. I just think of how I have been selfish and immature. I think that is what Tricia has always had trouble with me. I don't resent her, even though she treats me like crap. I figure I deserve it. I just take it. It helps to be like that because I don't fight her anymore. It is starting to confuse her, in a good way. She can see I haven't been drinking or getting together with my drinking buddies. I don't argue or complain about stuff. So she sees I'm different, but she is still so angry about the kids and everything. I don't know if she will ever forgive me for that, and I don't ask for it. I don't know if I will ever forgive myself.

"Things with the kids are different. I am absolutely all in on everything I can do to be a good father. And I don't mean the Disney World stuff. I mean just every time I get with them, paying attention to them. Listening to them and interested in what they are interested in. And correcting them, too. I actually think I have become a pretty good father. That's the thing that means the most to me. I take pride in that. I have a lot to do for them now. Evie has her exercises to do. Jack is messed up from the fire, scared to go to sleep, and having nightmares. I'm real patient about that because that is my doing. I never get upset with him for it. I'm pretty amazed, really, that I can so easily get through all that at night with him. Before I would have been so frustrated. I was selfish that way but not anymore…a hell of a way to become a better man. If I was this guy before, me and Tricia would be good. But like they say in AA, just focus on what you can change. That's maybe the biggest thing I got from AA.

"You know, I go to church with my folks. They tried for years to get me to go. Then they gave up. Then one day, I said, 'I'm going with you.' I just go. I don't know what to believe about it all yet, but it seems like a good thing. I guess I'm waiting to see what happens, but it seems like it fits with the new me. I've gotten involved with some of the mission stuff, the volunteering for things. I like being with these church guys, and a couple of them have really been good to me and have spent time with me. Maybe it's because they know my folks, but they have been very encouraging, and one guy I met at AA, too. I don't think I have had friends like that for a long time, maybe not since high school or maybe never, actually. I have never talked with anyone like that, so it has helped to talk some things out and get straight on what I'm really doing.

"But the strangest thing, maybe, is that I've been volunteering at a homeless shelter some nights. I don't want to sound great or anything, because I always thought those people were kind of a drag on society and whatnot, but I am much more understanding than I was before. It's strange. I guess I've started seeing things differently. The fire and all, I am so ashamed about it, I just can't get on my high horse anymore. I think of myself as undeserving, and it's not a bad thing. Makes it so I appreciate more and am more grateful, I guess. So I treat people better. Isn't it weird I am going to the homeless shelter rather than hanging out at the pub with the guys? Those guys aren't bad guys, but they just don't fit for me now.

"So, that's what's happening—a mess but with some good parts. There is a financial mess, a divorce for sure, Evie and Jack and all that they will need to get better. The hell I have put Tricia through and the hell I get back from her. But I am really more at peace than I have been before. I haven't gotten the plastic surgery. It's not a punishment or anything. I think it's just a reminder. I want to make sure I have this reminder. Maybe some day I won't need it, but right now, I'm not going to risk it.

"Sometimes I wonder where I would be if all this hadn't happened. Maybe I would have figured these things out. Maybe not. I don't know. But this has humbled me. I think that is what this did. Made me think different about myself. I just could not think the old selfish ways again. This put a big block to that. I just find it impossible to go back to that. I can't be grateful for that fire and what it did to my kids. I'm just grateful that I'm thinking right, got the right people around me, and doing right. I figure if I keep that up, my life will be all right."

Now that you have read this workbook, engaged in the exercises, and learned about posttraumatic growth, we hope you can not only find inspiration in this story but also go back through it and see the different kinds of growth Ryan describes and how this growth may have happened in his situation. You will notice core belief change, expert companionship, and a sense of mission now in his life. Applying these things to your own life is a challenge, but the pathway is there, and the rewards are great.

Congratulations on working your way through this workbook. You can now see that you have been living out your own compelling story with trauma as a turning point for changes in your life. You have reconsidered what you were like before trauma and what you have been becoming in its aftermath. Most importantly, you have now considered the possibility of who you may become. Your story is unfolding, and you are guiding the direction of it, although events can change this narrative quickly. But events do not need to dislodge the core beliefs and new identities that you've been establishing. Since these changes are built on principles of living that are growth-oriented responses to the greatest of challenges—pain, fear, and loss—you will be able to face future seismic events with greater resilience.

We also hope that by following the path laid out in this workbook, you will forge stronger interpersonal connections. We have encouraged you to accept assistance from expert companions, and you may also find meaning and sense of purpose in making it one of your missions to become an expert companion yourself.

We wish you the best on your path toward posttraumatic growth and invite you to make use of the resources available to you on our website: http://www.traumaand growth.com.

Suggested Reading

Resources for Trauma Survivors and Expert Companions

Mind-Body Workbook for PTSD: A 10-Week Program for Healing After Trauma, by S. H. Block and C. Bryant Block, 2010. Oakland, CA: New Harbinger Publications.

The Mindfulness-Based Emotional Balance Workbook: An Eight-Week Program for Improved Emotion Regulation and Resilience, by M. Cullen and G. Brito Pons, 2015. Oakland, CA: New Harbinger Publications.

Retelling the Stories of Our Lives: Everyday Narrative Therapy to Draw Inspiration and Transform Experience, by D. Denborough, 2014. New York: W. W. Norton and Co.

The Mindful Path to Self-Compassion: Freeing Yourself from Destructive Thoughts and Emotions, by C. K. Germer, 2009. New York: Guilford Press.

Surviving Survival: The Art and Science of Resilience, by L. Gonzales, 2012. New York: W. W. Norton and Co.

Bouncing Forward: Transforming Bad Breaks into Breakthroughs, by M. Haas, 2015. New York: Atria/Enliven Books.

What Doesn't Kill Us: The New Psychology of Posttraumatic Growth, by S. Joseph. 2011. New York: Basic Books.

Taking Control of Anxiety: Small Steps for Getting the Best of Worry, Stress, and Fear, by B. A. Moore, 2014. Washington, DC: American Psychological Association.

Wheels Down: Adjusting to Life After Deployment, by B. A. Moore and C. H. Kennedy, 2011. Washington, DC: American Psychological Association.

Upside: The New Science of Posttraumatic Growth, by J. Rendon, 2015. New York: Touchstone.

Step Out of Your Story: Writing Exercises to Reframe and Transform Your Life, by K. Schneiderman, 2015. Novato, CA: New World Library.

The PTSD Workbook: Simple, Effective Techniques for Overcoming Traumatic Stress Symptoms, 2nd edition, by M. B. Williams and S. Poijula, 2013. Oakland, CA: New Harbinger Publications.

When Someone You Love Suffers from Posttraumatic Stress: What to Expect and What You Can Do, by C. Zayfert and J. C. DeViva, 2011. New York: Guilford Press.

Resilience: Why Things Bounce Back, by A. Zolli and A. M. Healy, 2012. New York: Free Press.

Professional Resources

Stress, Trauma, and Posttraumatic Growth: Social Context, Environment, and Identities, by R. Berger, 2015. New York: Routledge/Taylor and Francis Group.

Handbook of Posttraumatic Growth: Research and Practice, edited by L. G. Calhoun and R. G. Tedeschi, 2006. New York: Routledge/Taylor and Francis Group.

Posttraumatic Growth in Clinical Practice, by L. G. Calhoun and R. G. Tedeschi, 2013. New York: Routledge/Taylor and Francis Group.

Trauma and the Therapeutic Relationship: Approaches to Process and Practice, by D. Murphy and S. Joseph, 2013. New York: Palgrave Macmillan.

Meaning Reconstruction and the Experience of Loss, edited by R. A. Neimeyer, 2001. Washington DC: American Psychological Association.

Life After Loss: Contemporary Grief Counseling and Therapy, by J. Rainer, 2013. Eau Claire, WI: PESI Publishing and Media.

Helping Bereaved Parents: A Clinician's Guide, by R. G. Tedeschi and L. G. Calhoun. 2003. New York: Routledge/Taylor and Francis Group.

Trauma and Transformation: Growing in the Aftermath of Suffering, by R. G. Tedeschi and L. G. Calhoun, 1995. Thousand Oaks, CA: Sage Publications.

References

American Psychiatric Association. 2013. *Diagnostic and Statistical Manual of Mental Disorders (DSM-5)*. 5th ed. Washington, DC: American Psychiatric Association.

Calhoun, L. G., and R. G. Tedeschi, eds. 2006. *Handbook of Posttraumatic Growth: Research and Practice*. New York: Routledge.

Cann, A., L. G. Calhoun, R. G. Tedeschi, R. P. Kilmer, V. Gil-Rivas, T. Vishnevsky, and S. C. Danhauer. 2009. "The Core Beliefs Inventory: A Brief Measure of Disruption in the Assumptive World." *Anxiety, Stress and Coping* 23 (1) 19–34.

Cann, A., L. G. Calhoun, R. G. Tedeschi, K. N. Triplett, T. Vishnevsky, and C. M. Lindstrom. 2011. "Assessing Posttraumatic Cognitive Processes: The Event Related Rumination Inventory." *Anxiety, Stress, and Coping* 24 (2): 137–56.

Freeman, A., and S. M. Freeman. 2009. "Vulnerability Factors: Raising and Lowering the Threshold for Response." In *Living and Surviving in Harm's Way: A Psychological Treatment Handbook for Pre- and Post-Deployment of Military Personnel*, edited by S. M. Freeman, B. A. Moore, A. Freeman. New York: Routledge/Taylor and Francis Group.

Johnson, H., and A. Thompson. 2008. "The Development and Maintenance of Post-Traumatic Stress Disorder (PTSD) in Civilian Adult Survivors of War Trauma and Torture: A Review." *Clinical Psychology Review* 28 (1): 36–47.

Kilpatrick, D. G., H. S. Resnick, M. E. Milanak, M. W. Miller, K. M. Keyes, and M. J. Friedman. 2013. "National Estimates of Exposure to Traumatic Events and PTSD Prevalence Using DSM-IV and DSM-5 Criteria." *Journal of Traumatic Stress* 26 (5): 537–47.

Mills, K. L., A. C. McFarlane, T. Slade, M. Creamer, D. Silove, M. Teesson, and R. Bryant. 2011. "Assessing the Prevalence of Trauma Exposure in Epidemiological Surveys." *Australian and New Zealand Journal of Psychiatry* 45 (5): 407–15.

Nebraska Department of Veterans' Affairs. 2007. "Post-Traumatic Stress Disorder." http://www.ptsd.ne.gov/what-is-ptsd.html.

Norris, F. H. 1992. "Epidemiology of Trauma: Frequency and Impact of Different Potentially Traumatic Events on Different Demographic Groups." *Journal of Consulting and Clinical Psychology* 60 (3): 409–18.

Tedeschi, R. G., and L. G. Calhoun. 1996. "The Posttraumatic Growth Inventory: Measuring the Positive Legacy of Trauma." *Journal of Traumatic Stress* 9 (3): 455–71.

Richard G. Tedeschi, PhD, is professor of psychology at the University of North Carolina at Charlotte, and a licensed psychologist in practice for over thirty-five years. He helped originate the concept of posttraumatic growth (PTG), and has published many academic books and articles on the subject. Tedeschi has consulted with the US Army and many other institutions to train professionals in growth-oriented practice.

Bret A. Moore, PsyD, ABPP, is a prescribing psychologist and board-certified clinical psychologist in San Antonio, TX. He is a former active-duty Army psychologist and two-tour veteran of Iraq. Moore is the author and editor of fifteen books and has authored dozens of book chapters, scientific papers, and popular press articles. His views on clinical psychology have been quoted in *USA Today*, *The New York Times*, and *The Boston Globe*, and on CNN and Fox News. He has appeared on NPR, the BBC, and CBC.

Real change *is* possible

For more than forty-five years, New Harbinger has published proven-effective self-help books and pioneering workbooks to help readers of all ages and backgrounds improve mental health and well-being, and achieve lasting personal growth. In addition, our spirituality books offer profound guidance for deepening awareness and cultivating healing, self-discovery, and fulfillment.

Founded by psychologist Matthew McKay and Patrick Fanning, New Harbinger is proud to be an independent, employee-owned company. Our books reflect our core values of integrity, innovation, commitment, sustainability, compassion, and trust. Written by leaders in the field and recommended by therapists worldwide, New Harbinger books are practical, accessible, and provide real tools for real change.

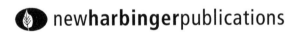 **newharbinger**publications

MORE BOOKS *from*
NEW HARBINGER PUBLICATIONS

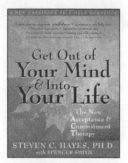

GET OUT OF YOUR MIND & INTO YOUR LIFE
The New Acceptance & Commitment Therapy
ISBN: 978-1572244252 / US $21.95

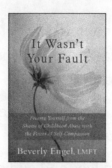

IT WASN'T YOUR FAULT
Freeing Yourself from the Shame of Childhood Abuse with the Power of Self-Compassion
ISBN: 978-1626250994 / US $16.95

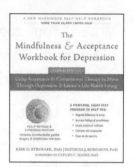

THE MINDFULNESS & ACCEPTANCE WORKBOOK FOR DEPRESSION, SECOND EDITION
Using Acceptance & Commitment Therapy to Move Through Depression & Create a Life Worth Living
ISBN: 978-1626258457 / US $24.95

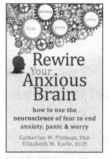

REWIRE YOUR ANXIOUS BRAIN
How to Use the Neuroscience of Fear to End Anxiety, Panic & Worry
ISBN: 978-1626251137 / US $16.95

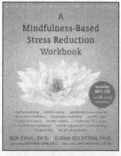

A MINDFULNESS-BASED STRESS REDUCTION WORKBOOK
ISBN: 978-1572247086 / US $24.95

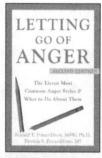

LETTING GO OF ANGER, SECOND EDITION
The Eleven Most Common Anger Styles & What to Do About Them
ISBN: 978-1572244481 / US $16.95

newharbingerpublications
1-800-748-6273 / newharbinger.com

(VISA, MC, AMEX / prices subject to change without notice)

Follow Us

Don't miss out on new books in the subjects that interest you.
Sign up for our **Book Alerts** at **newharbinger.com/bookalerts**

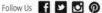

ARE YOU SEEKING A CBT THERAPIST?
The Association for Behavioral & Cognitive Therapies (ABCT) Find-a-Therapist service offers a list of therapists schooled in CBT techniques. Therapists listed are licensed professionals who have met the membership requirements of ABCT & who have chosen to appear in the directory.
Please visit www.abct.org & click on *Find a Therapist*.

Register your **new harbinger** titles for additional benefits!

When you register your **new harbinger** title—purchased in any format, from any source—you get access to benefits like the following:

- Downloadable accessories like printable worksheets and extra content

- Instructional videos and audio files

- Information about updates, corrections, and new editions

Not every title has accessories, but we're adding new material all the time.

Access free accessories in 3 easy steps:

1. Sign in at NewHarbinger.com (or **register** to create an account).

2. Click on **register a book**. Search for your title and click the **register** button when it appears.

3. Click on the **book cover or title** to go to its details page. Click on **accessories** to view and access files.

That's all there is to it!

If you need help, visit:

NewHarbinger.com/accessories

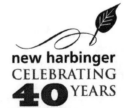

new harbinger
CELEBRATING
40 YEARS